RENAL AND UROLOGIC DISORDERS

URINARY TRACT INFECTIONS

EPIDEMIOLOGY, PATHOGENESIS AND PREVENTION

RENAL AND UROLOGIC DISORDERS

Additional books in this series can be found on Nova's website
under the Series tab.

Additional e-books in this series can be found on Nova's website
under the e-book tab.

RENAL AND UROLOGIC DISORDERS

URINARY TRACT INFECTIONS

EPIDEMIOLOGY, PATHOGENESIS AND PREVENTION

KRISTEN E. MURRELL
EDITOR

New York

For permission to use material from this book please contact us:
Telephone 631-231-7269; Fax 631-231-8175
Web Site: http://www.novapublishers.com

Library of Congress Cataloging-in-Publication Data

ISBN: 978-1-63117-180-2

Library of Congress Control Number: 2014930034

Published by Nova Science Publishers, Inc. † New York

Contents

Preface

Urinary tract infections (UTI) are one of the most common bacterial infections seen. Episodes of UTI can effectively be treated with antibiotics, often given on an empirical basis. In this book, the authors present current research in UTI's. Topics discussed in this compilation include the antibiotic and non-antibiotic methods of prophylaxis for recurrent UTI's; UTI's in children; virulence factors of uropathogenic Escherichia coli and their role in development of UTI's; and the treatment for UTI's due to multidrug-resistant bacteria.

Chapter 1 - Urinary tract infections (UTIs) are one of the most common bacterial infections seen. Episodes of UTI can effectively be treated with antibiotics, often given on an empirical basis. For patients with recurrent UTIs, i.e., patients with at least 3 UTIs within a period of 12 months, antibiotic prophylaxis has been shown to reduce the number of UTI episodes.

However, this poses a high selective antibiotic pressure on the bacteria causing the UTIs, i.e., the uropathogens, in this patient population. For this reason, several non-antibiotic alternatives for the prophylaxis of UTIs have been developed in order to reduce the antibiotic load to which uropathogens are exposed. In this chapter we review the current options, antibiotic as well as non-antibiotic alternatives, for the prevention of rUTIs. In summary, antibiotic alternatives to the continuous low-dose antibiotic prophylaxis, such as self-treatment and post-coital prophylaxis, show promising results, although these regimens will not be applicable to all women with rUTI. The effectiveness of most non-antibiotic alternatives remains inconclusive, mainly because of the lack of trials among human subjects or inconsistency in the type and dosage used in clinical trials. We opt for consensus on the specific regimen that needs evaluation for each non-antibiotic group, which makes powerful meta-analyses possible. Hereby, the actual value of specific non-antibiotic options could be assessed, increasing the chance of incorporating an effective non-antibiotic option in clinical guidelines. Subsequently, the substantial antibiotic use among women with rUTI will be lowered, resulting in a better control of antibiotic resistance.

Chapter 2 – Urinary tract infections (UTI) are among the most common bacterial infections in childhood. Its general incidence varies according to age and gender, but it is difficult to establish accurately because of the heterogeneity in UTI's definition, the population included, and the studies design and methodology.

In addition, symptoms in young children are frequently nonspecific. Some studies have shown a higher incidence of UTI in males than females during the first months of life, but this relation is reversed thereafter.

The estimated incidence in girls varies from 2.1% to 11.3%, and in boys from 1.0% to 3.6%, depending on age. As for the race, the available data suggests that the incidence of UTI is lower in African Americans as compared to White, Hispanic and Asian children.

The prevalence of acute pyelonephritis (APN) defined clinically (fever > 38.5°C, and C reactive protein > 20 mg/L) in pediatric patients with UTI is around 59% in boys and 32% in girls. Some studies using renal scintigraphy (DMSA) found a prevalence of APN in children with febrile UTI of 50-80%, while renal parenchymal inflammation was rarely found in lower tract infections. Although uncommon in children, renal abscesses are potential serious complications of UTI, but their incidence is also imprecisely known.

The most frequent pathogen involved in ascending infections is Escherichia coli, but Staphylococcus aureus is common after hematogenous dissemination. Acute focal bacterial nephritis is also rare in infancy although it could be an under-diagnosed condition.

The prevalence of vesicoureteral reflux (VUR) in the general population is around 1-3%, but in pediatric patients with UTI it ranges from 18% to 38%, and it is bilateral in half of the cases. Other nephro-urological structural anomalies that may contribute to the UTI pathogenesis are hydronephrosis and renal system duplication, present in 2.5-7.5% and 6-7% of cases, respectively.

The main etiological agent in childhood's UTI is Escherichia coli (70-90%). However, other bacteria should also be considered in children previously exposed to antibiotics, and among those hospitalized or with nephro-urological anomalies.

The infection usually starts with the perianal colonization by intestinal bacteria, with posterior invasion of the urethra, and ascending progression to other areas of the nephro-urological system.

While individual and genetic predisposition to UTI are recognized, the main factor favoring bacterial colonization and its progression to the upper urinary tract is the ability of the microorganisms to adhere to uroepithelial cells by pili or fimbriae (mainly the type 2 or P). This mechanism is favored by urinary stasis secondary to VUR and by obstructive processes that allow bacterial replication.

Given that bad voiding habits (infrequent emptying) and constipation are associated with an increased incidence of UTI, its correction, together with an increase in fluid intake may be beneficial to prevent bacterial multiplication and their migration to the upper urinary tract regions. Antibiotic prophylaxis should be considered in children with severe VUR (grades IV and V), genitourinary anomalies and recurrent infections. High-risk boys may also benefit from circumcision.

Chapter 3 – Uropathogenic *Escherichia coli* (UPEC) are the major etiological agent of urinary tract infections (UTIs). UPEC differ from non-pathogenic *E. coli* by the presence of virulence factors which enable these bacteria to colonize uroepithelial cells and to establish a UTI. These include a range of adherence factors, toxins, iron uptake systems, and capsules. Evolutionary influences on the acquisition and main role of virulence genes amongst *E. coli* are widely debated, with some research holding that the prevalence of strains with virulence genes increases the likelihood of infection, whereas other believe that virulence genes provide a selective advantage for infection of extraintestinal sites. UPEC strains causing UTI are often found among the faecal flora of the host. The presence and persistence of these strains in the gastrointestinal (GI) tract is facilitated by their adhesion to intestinal epithelial cells. This may serve as a source for the development of UTI if their numbers increases and dominate the *E. coli* population of the GI tract in the host.

Chapter 4 – Inappropriate use of antibiotics together with evolving resistance of bacteria has increased the prevalence of infections due to multidrug-resistant (MDR) bacteria worldwide over the past few decades. Urinary tract infections are amongst the most common infectious diseases affected by the increasing burden of antibiotic resistance. Selection of appropriate empiric and definite antibiotic therapy for urinary tract infection (UTI) has become more challenging for healthcare providers resulting in delay in appropriate therapy. Several factors need to be taken into account for antibiotic selection. These include patient's characteristics, history of prior UTI treatment, previous antibiotic exposure and local antibiotic resistance pattern. Some of the uropathogenic MDR bacteria that are threats for healthcare system include gram-positive MDR bacteria, such as methicillin-resistant *Staphylococcus aureus* and vancomycin-resistant enterococci and gram-negative MDR bacteria, such as the Enterobacteriaceae, *Pseudomonas aeruginosa* and *Acinetobacter baumannii*. Urinary tract infections due to these organisms require early appropriate antibiotic treatment to prevent morbidity and mortality. In some cases, novel methods of antibiotic administration including combination therapy and prolonged infusion therapy may be required. In complicated cases, combined surgical interventions are needed along with antibiotic therapy. In addition, infection control measures are necessary to prevent further transmission of these MDR bacteria between patients and within a hospital. This chapter reviews the epidemiology of MDR bacteria, appropriate empiric and definite treatments and adjunctive measures and strategies to manage UTIs caused by the MDR bacteria.

In: Urinary Tract Infections
Editor: Kristen E. Murrell
ISBN: 978-1-63117-180-2

Chapter 1

Antibiotic and Non-Antibiotic Methods of Prophylaxis for Recurrent Urinary Tract Infections

Casper D. J. den Heijer[1,*] *and Ellen E. Stobberingh*[2]
[1]Department of Medical Microbiology, Maastricht University Medical Centre/CAPHRI, Maastricht, The Netherlands
[2]National Institute for Public Health and the Environment, Centre for Infectious Disease Control Netherlands (CIb), Bilthoven, The Netherlands

Abstract

Urinary tract infections (UTIs) are one of the most common bacterial infections seen. Episodes of UTI can effectively be treated with antibiotics, often given on an empirical basis. For patients with recurrent UTIs, i.e., patients with at least 3 UTIs within a period of 12 months, antibiotic prophylaxis has been shown to reduce the number of UTI episodes.

* Corresponding author: Dr. C. D. J. den Heijer, Maastricht University Medical Centre, Department of Medical Microbiology, PO Box 5800, 6202AZ Maastricht, The Netherlands. Phone: +31-43-3876647, Fax: +31-43-3876643, E-mail: casper.den.heijer@mumc.nl.

However, this poses a high selective antibiotic pressure on the bacteria causing the UTIs, i.e., the uropathogens, in this patient population. For this reason, several non-antibiotic alternatives for the prophylaxis of UTIs have been developed in order to reduce the antibiotic load to which uropathogens are exposed. In this chapter we review the current options, antibiotic as well as non-antibiotic alternatives, for the prevention of rUTIs. In summary, antibiotic alternatives to the continuous low-dose antibiotic prophylaxis, such as self-treatment and post-coital prophylaxis, show promising results, although these regimens will not be applicable to all women with rUTI. The effectiveness of most non-antibiotic alternatives remains inconclusive, mainly because of the lack of trials among human subjects or inconsistency in the type and dosage used in clinical trials. We opt for consensus on the specific regimen that needs evaluation for each non-antibiotic group, which makes powerful meta-analyses possible. Hereby, the actual value of specific non-antibiotic options could be assessed, increasing the chance of incorporating an effective non-antibiotic option in clinical guidelines. Subsequently, the substantial antibiotic use among women with rUTI will be lowered, resulting in a better control of antibiotic resistance.

Introduction

Urinary tract infections (UTIs) are one of the most common bacterial infections seen, which predominantly affect women. It has been estimated that approximately 50% of all women experience at least one episode of UTI during their lifetime. [1]

In addition, almost half of all women with an initial UTI, develops a recurrence within one year. [2]

For patients with recurrent UTIs (rUTIs), i.e., patients with at least three UTIs within a period of 12 months, actions can be undertaken to prevent a new recurrence. After the exclusion of co-morbidities that can be related to the rUTIs (e.g., pelvic organ prolapse), the clinician can discuss whether the UTIs coincide with specific behaviours (e.g., sexual intercourse, or the use of spermicide-containing products) with the patient. [3, 4] If this is the case, behavioural changes can be helpful in the prevention of the rUTIs, for example voiding after sexual intercourse.

If this approach cannot solve the problem, antibiotic prophylaxis has shown to reduce the number of UTI episodes. [5] However, this poses a highly selective antibiotic pressure on the bacteria causing the UTIs in this patient population, of which *Escherichia coli* is the most commonly encountered. [4]

For this reason, several non-antibiotic alternatives for the prophylaxis of rUTIs have been developed in order to reduce the antibiotic load to which uropathogens are exposed.

In this chapter we will review the current options, antibiotic as well as non-antibiotic, for the prevention of rUTIs. Our aim was not to be exhaustive, but to provide the reader a general overview of most of the currently available alternatives in the prophylaxis of rUTI. The focus will be on prophylactic regimens that are applicable to non-pregnant adult women.

Antibiotic Prophylaxis

The effectiveness of long-term low-dose antibiotic prophylaxis of rUTI has long been established. [6] This evidence was supported by a Cochrane review in 2004, including ten trials with 430 women in which 6-12 months of antibiotic prophylaxis was compared to placebo. [5] The Cochrane meta-analysis showed that the number of UTI recurrences ranged from 0 to 0.9 in the antibiotic group compared with a range of 0.8 to 3.6 in the placebo group. However, patients receiving antibiotics were more likely to experience side effects, such as vaginal and oral candidiasis and gastrointestinal symptoms.

Apart from continuous prophylaxis, also other regimens have been evaluated. In women who have shown to adequately identify their UTI, self-treatment can be an option. [7] In this case, it is important that women receive clear instructions when they should contact their clinician in order to prevent alarming situations. [3] Post-coital prophylaxis can be considered in women in whom the UTI is clearly associated with sexual intercourse. [8]

These alternative regimens have been compared with the continuous antibiotic prophylactic approach. In a recent randomized controlled trial (RCT) among postmenopausal women with rUTI, patient-initiated single-dose treatment was compared with continuous low-dose antibiotic prophylaxis. [9] Here it was reported that both regimens reduced the number of UTI recurrences significantly compared with the 12 months preceding the trial. In addition, the self-treatment group showed less gastrointestinal adverse events than the continuous group (9.1% versus 30.0%, respectively).

Melekos et al. evaluated the efficacy of daily prophylactic treatment versus post-coital antibiotic prophylaxis in 135 sexually active, premenopausal women. [8] Similar to the findings in the above mentioned RCT, they found significant reductions in UTI recurrences compared with the pre-study year for both regimens.

Both the self-treatment and post-coital regimens have the benefit of reducing the antimicrobial load to which the patients are exposed. [8, 10] The effects of long-term antibiotic administration on the patients microbiota have been demonstrated by Beerepoot et al. [11] After the use of trimethoprim/ sulfamethoxazole (TMP/SMZ, 480mg once daily) for one month, they reported that 86.3% of the fecal and 90.5% of urinary *E. coli* isolates were TMP/SMZ-resistant compared with 23.7% and 28.1% in the non-antibiotic group, respectively. In general, the clinical relevance of antibiotic resistance has been shown by an increase in morbidity and mortality, probably due to a delay in effective treatment. [12, 13]

For this reason, the choice of the antibiotic to use in the prophylactic regimen is of importance. Because of the good safety profile and low costs, TMP/SMZ has long been considered the first choice for UTI treatment (and prophylaxis) in many countries. [7, 14] However, the appropriateness of this drug in the UTI treatment regimen has been questioned, because of the report of increasing levels of resistance. [15-17] Gupta et al. proposed that if *E. coli* antibiotic resistance exceeds 20%, this antibiotic should not be prescribed empirically. [18] This threshold can be helpful to decide whether or not TMP/ SMZ is still an appropriate empirical choice in the treatment and prevention of UTI per country and setting.

Fluoroquinolones can accurately treat UTIs, but are generally considered second-line treatment options in order to preserve their effectiveness. At this moment, levels of fluoroquinolone *E. coli* resistance are, in general, lower than that of TMP/SMX, but previous reports have shown that fluoroquinolone resistance can quickly arise after its (clinical) use. [19]

Nitrofurantoin has been used for decades in the treatment of UTIs without a significant increase in resistance. The only drawback of this drug are the serious adverse events that have been reported, although very rarely, after long-term exposure, including (sub)acute and chronic pulmonary reactions, chronic hepatitis and neuropathy. [7] These considerations make this drug, at the least, suitable for the non-continuous prophylactic regimens.

Finally, a single-dose fosfomycin has proven to be effective in treating an uncomplicated UTI without the cost of increasing levels of resistance. [20] In addition, fosfomycin has been shown to be effective against multidrug-resistant (e.g., extended-spectrum beta-lactamase (ESBL)-producing bacteria) and no serious side effects have been reported yet. [21] In this way, fosfomycin can be an appropriate treatment option, although its value in long-term prophylactic treatment has to be established yet.

Next to the considerations of the appropriateness of an antibiotic per country and setting, the prophylactic regimen should, ideally, be determined on a per-patient basis. It has been shown that the most recent *E. coli* antibiotic susceptibility patterns are predictive for the *E. coli* strain involved in UTI. [22, 23]

Therefore, on the patient-level, the antibiotic of choice should depend on the most recently available antibiotic resistance pattern, together with the patient's history of allergies or other adverse reactions to previous antibiotic challenges.

In addition, the patient's willingness to use antibiotics for a relatively long period should be discussed by the clinician. [24]

Non-Antibiotic Prophylaxis

Apart from the negative effects on the patient's own microbiotia (e.g., increasing antibiotic resistance), disadvantages of antibiotic prophylaxis include the interaction with other drugs including contraceptives, and antibiotic-induced diarrhoea. [7] In addition, the prophylactic effect seems short-lived, because the 2004 Cochrane review reported that once the antibiotic prophylaxis is stopped, the rate of UTI recurrences returns to the level of the placebo group. [5]

For these reasons, non-antibiotic prophylactic options have been investigated. In order to accurately understand the different non-antibiotic regimens, sufficient knowledge on UTI pathogenesis is necessary. For this reason, we shall briefly address the onset of UTIs.

It is known that UTIs result from the entry of uropathogens into the urinary tract, with *Escherichia coli* most regularly involved. The most common route is via the urethra by bacteria that originate in the rectal flora (the ascending route). Vaginal colonization by uropathogens is considered to be a prerequisite prior to bladder infection via this route.

Whether an infection actually occurs, is mainly determined by whether the causative pathogen can adhere to the epithelial cells in the bladder of the host. [25, 26] Therefore, the adherence to uroepithelial cells is an important target for most types of non-antibiotic profylaxes.

In the following sections we will describe the mode of action, effectiveness and reported side effects of the major non-antibiotic prophylaxis groups.

Cranberries

In the past, it was hypothesized that cranberries can prevent UTIs via lowering the urine pH, via the ingredient quinic acid which causes large amounts of hippuric acid to be excreted. [27] However, this mechanism does not seem plausible, because people are not able to consume sufficient volumes of cranberry juice to establish an acidic, bacteriostatic environment in the bladder. [28] Research has shown that a specific compound of cranberries, i.e., proanthocyanidin (PAC), plays a role in the inhibition of the binding of the P-fimbriae of uropathogens, which prevents the bacteria from entering the bladder cell and causing the infection. [28] The recent, updated Cochrane review by Jepson et al. included four studies that compared cranberry products with placebo. [29-32] The meta-analysis showed a non-significant reduced risk of the cranberry treatment (relative risk (RR) 0.74, 95% confidence interval (CI) 0.42 to 1.31) with heterogeneity between the studies. The most recent, and largest, study [32] showed no benefit of cranberry treatment, whereas the three older, smaller studies were more optimistic about the effectiveness of cranberries. Reasons for this discrepancy were discussed to be the difference in power and the difference in threshold used to determine a UTI. Furthermore, the amount of PAC, the active ingredient in cranberries, was only given in the most recent study, making differences in PAC concentration a possible additional factor to explain the discordant outcomes. Interestingly, from the pooled analysis of two studies that compared cranberry juice with antibiotic prophylaxis, it could be concluded that antibiotics are not superior to cranberries (RR 1.31, 95% CI 0.85 to 2.02). [27] However, apart from the apparent limited effectiveness, most studies reported high withdrawal rates in the cranberry group, because large proportions of patients found it inconvenient to consume cranberry juice over such a long period. These observations make cranberries in juice form currently not a suitable option in the prevention of rUTIs. However, different formulations (tablets, capsules) have only rarely been used in RCTs, even less with the appropriate dosage of PACs, so these could be further investigated in women with rUTI.

Lactobacilli

Another group that has been hypothesized to be able to prevent rUTIs, is the hydrogen peroxide-producing lactobacillus, which works by restoring the normal (acidic) vaginal microbiota in women with rUTI.

This mechanism is evident in postmenopausal women, with postmenopausal reductions in estrogen causing lactobacil levels to drop. However, even in premenopausal women prone to rUTIs, a change in the vaginal microbiota has been shown, with depletion of lactobacilli. [33]

From the many different strains of lactobacilli, *Lacobacillus rhamnosus* GR-1 and *L. reuteri* RC-14 have been assumed to be the most effective for the prevention of rUTI. [34] Beerepoot et al. evaluated capsules with these lactobacil strains in 252 postmenopausal women in a randomized, double-blind, non-inferiority trial, with TMP/SMZ prophylaxis as the standard treatment. There was a between-treatment difference of 0.4 UTIs per year (95% CI, -0.4 to 1.5) in favour of the antibiotic treatment, from which non-inferiority could not be concluded. [35] Serious adverse events were not significantly different between the two groups. The major disadvantage of the antibiotic group was the increase of *E. coli* resistance to TMP/SMZ, within one month after the start of antibiotic treatment.

Studies looking at other regimens include amongst others an older study (1995), which showed that vaginally administered prophylaxis of the combination of *L. rhamnosus* GR-1 and *L. reuteri* B-54 once weekly reduced rUTIs in premenopausal women from 6.0 to 1.6 UTIs per year. [36]

Another study, including 100 premenopausal women, used a product called Lactin-V, which is an intravaginal probiotic composed of *L. crispatus* CTV-05. [33] In comparison with placebo, there was a non-significant decrease in the number of UTIs during 10 weeks of follow-up (RR 0.5, 95% CI: 0.2 to 1.2). The women in the Lactin-V group who reached a high-level of colonization of *L. crispatus* showed a significant reduction compared with those who did not. [33] It would be of interest to further analyse the factors that determined whether a woman reached a high-level of *L. crispatus* CTV-05 colonization or not.

Serious adverse events (e.g., bacteraemia) in patients receiving lactobacilli have only been described in patients having complicated conditions, such as those who are immunocompromised or premature infants. [37] Apart from these patients, no serious side effects have been reported so far.

With this overview, it remains inconclusive whether lactobacilli can effectively prevent rUTI, because of the diversity of strains used in the studies and the different dosing regimens, which is in line with a 2008 review on this topic. [37]

Therefore, there is an urgent need for consensus on the type and dosage of lactobacil strains to use, in order to accurately evaluate the value of lactobacilli in preventing rUTIs.

Estrogen Administration

As previously mentioned, estrogen is important for the proliferation of lactobacilli in the vaginal epithelium, thereby reducing the pH, which prevents vaginal colonization with Enterobacteriaceae. [38] Next to the supplementation of lactobacilli, estrogen administration has been evaluated in preventing rUTIs.

Besides the influence on the vaginal microbiota, a recently published study looked at the specific effects of estrogens on the bladder epithelium. [39] This revealed that estrogens promote the expression of antimicrobial peptides and strengthen intercellular junctions, thereby preventing the loss of many superficial cells during infection.

On the other hand, it was shown that estrogen promotes a higher number of bacteria to be taken up by the urothelial cells, thus showing arguments pro and contra the preventive effect of estrogen administration.

There are several methods of estrogen administration: oral, vaginal cream, vaginal tablets, vaginal ring and vaginal pessaries. [40] Oral supplementation has the disadvantage of being passed through the liver where estrogen is partially metabolized, which necessitates much higher doses orally compared with vaginal administrations. [38]

In a Cochrane review by Perrotta et al. in 2008, comparing women receiving oral estrogens or placebo, a similar proportion had a UTI after the intervention (RR 1.08, 95% CI 0.88 to 1.33). [40] For vaginal applications, there was a beneficial effect compared with placebo in two studies. [41, 42]

When Perrotta et al. compared the different forms of applications between studies, it appeared that vaginal cream had the best results in estrogen versus antibiotic studies.

However, it was noted that in the study using vaginal cream, a high number of UTIs were experienced in the antibiotic group, thereby exaggerating the effect of the estrogen therapy.

In addition, several side effects were reported by women using the cream, including vaginal itching, burning and, less regularly, spotting. [40] It was advised that vaginal creams are an option in the outpatient setting, whereas vaginal rings and pessaries could be more suitable in a nursing home situation, where patients often have more difficulty applying creams.

The increased knowledge on the working mechanism of estrogens in the bladder can help to further optimize the application of estrogens in the prevention of rUTI.

Colonization with a Non-Pathogenic *Escherichia coli* Strain

The non-virulent *E. coli* strain 83972 has been investigated thoroughly since it has been isolated from a schoolgirl who carried the strain for a 3-years period without loss of renal function or experiencing an episode of UTI. [43] The effectiveness of this non-pathogenic strain has been attributed to “bacterial interference”: by competition of nutrients and the production of toxic molecules, the urinary tract becomes less accessible for pathogenic strains. [44]

The reason for not causing symptoms of UTI was investigated by Lutay et al. who evaluated host gene expression *in vitro* after *E. coli* strain 83972 colonization and compared it with expressions after uropathogenic *E. coli* (UPEC) challenge. It appeared that strain 83972 downregulated RNA polymerase II–dependent transcription, while this transcription was upregulated by the UPEC strain. [45] These results imply that *E. coli* strain 83972 can alter the host immune response, resulting in a lack of UTI symptoms, thereby favouring its survival.

A placebo-controlled trial observed a significantly longer time period to a next episode of *E. coli* UTI when patients were colonized with strain 83972 compared to placebo. [46] In addition, few side effects were noted that were related to this intervention. However, there were difficulties in acquiring an asymptomatic bacteriuria (ASB) state with this strain in all recruited patients, which questions whether this approach is applicable to all patients with rUTI. Moreover, in few patients in whom ASB was reached, reinoculation was required, which can pose problems in the real-life setting where patients are less well monitored.

In addition, patients who were colonized did experience UTIs during follow-up and it was argued whether strain 83972 would not be able to cause a UTI itself after long-term carriage. [46]

Recently, the recombinant *E. coli* 83972::*lgtCE* strain has been developed, that binds to the P-fimbriae receptor on (virulent) *E. coli*, thereby inhibiting the attachment to kidney cells and thus preventing pyelonephritis. [47] In addition, it was shown in a mouse model that this modified strain could prevent urinary colonization in the bladder.

In conclusion, research on *E. coli* strain 83972 has given insights in the differences between ASB and pathogenic strains. Despite the fact that colonization with this strain can lead to difficulties in a non-experimental setting, the knowledge provided by these trials can result in new possibilities in preventing rUTIs.

Vaccines

E. coli is the pathogen most commonly encountered in UTIs and, therefore, vaccines developed to prevent UTIs are mainly targeted against this bacterium. Requirements for a vaccine include that it should be highly immunogenic and expressed by the bacterium during infection on its surface, in order to be picked-up and recognized by the host immune system. [48] Moreover, it should be pathogen-specific, because commensal *E. coli* should not be affected.

Initially, the scientific community showed interest in vaccines aimed at the bacterial lipopolysaccharides (LPS; including the O antigen) and the polysaccharide coat, also known as the capsule (K antigen). However, the lack of immunogenicity and specificity of these antigens limited the continued evaluation of these vaccines. [48]

A next, more promising category, are the formulas with whole or lysed parts of inactivated pathogens. The OM-89, which is a cocktail of membrane proteins from 18 uropathogenic *E. coli* strains, showed promising results in a recent meta-analysis. [24] This analysis included 4 trials comparing this formula with placebo: the proportion of patients with at least one UTI during follow-up was significantly lower in the OM-89 group (RR 0.61, 95% CI 0.48 to 0.78) and adverse events were comparable to placebo. One potential problem could be that this capsule needs to be taken for a period of 90 days (once daily), and this relatively long period could lead to suboptimal patient compliance. [48]

In a retrospective observational study, Lorenzo-Gómez et al. evaluated the Uromune® vaccine, containing an inactivated bacterial cell suspension of specific strains of *Escherichia coli*, *Klebsiella pneumoniae*, *Proteus vulgaris*, and *Enterococcus faecalis*. [49] In 319 women with rUTI, this vaccine was compared with continuous TMP/SMZ prophylaxis. Results were in favour of the Uromune® vaccine, although the proportion of women with UTI during follow-up was very high in the TMP/SMZ group (94% after three months), thereby possibly exaggerating the Uromune® vaccine effect.

Adherence of bacterial cells to the host bladder cell are mediated by adhesins, of which fimbriae and pili are examples.

In this respect, the adhesin FimH, that plays an important role in *E. coli* binding to bladder epithelial cells, has been investigated. [48] Despite disappointing results of vaccines looking at this protein solely, a recent paper showed better results of FimH in combination with adjuvants in a mice model. [50]

Significantly higher immune responses were noted for the FimH-adjuvant vaccine compared with FimH alone and less colonization of *E. coli* was observed. These promising results require verification in trials involving human subjects.

Finally, metal ions are important for many processes in *E. coli*, in particular iron. Because of the limited iron availability in the human urogenital tract, *E. coli* have outer membrane iron compound receptors, that are capable of acquiring this metal from the host environment. [51] These receptors are good candidates for vaccine development, because they are externally located on the bacterium, present at the time of infection and common in pathogenic *E. coli* strains. From previous results it appears that multiple receptors need to be targeted to get an adequate response. [48] Moreover, it has been reported that the importance of iron-acquiring systems differ per location (kidney, bladder), which could make it possible to specifically target *E. coli* involved in pyelonephritis and cystitis, respectively. [52] More research needs to be conducted to further clarify these iron-uptake systems.

Overall, most of the addressed vaccine-targets give promising results, although further research is necessary to evaluate the effects *in vivo*. Because of the heterogeneity of *E. coli* strains, an effective vaccine would possibly require the incorporation of a combination of these mechanisms.

Conclusion

Although the effectiveness of continuous antibiotic prophylaxis to susceptible uropathogens is not being questioned, the quick emergence of antibiotic-resistant bacteria, in particular extended-spectrum beta-lactamase producers, shows the need for (non-)antibiotic alternatives.

With respect to the antibiotic treatment options, alternative regimens have been shown to be equally effective as the continuous prophylaxis, including self-treatment and post-coital prophylaxis, although these regimens will not be applicable to all women with rUTI.

The effectiveness of most non-antibiotic prophylactic options remains inconclusive, mainly because of the lack of trials among human subjects or inconsistency in the type and dosage used in clinical trials.

For this reason, we opt for consensus on the specific regimen that needs evaluation for each non-antibiotic group. In this way, powerful meta-analyses of studies with similar designs can be performed, thereby assessing the value of that specific non-antibiotic alternative.

When these analyses show beneficial results, chances increase that these non-antibiotic prophylatic regimens will be included in clinical guidelines. Subsequently, the substantial antibiotic use among women with rUTI will be lowered, resulting in a better control of antibiotic resistance.

References

[1] Foxman, B. Epidemiology of urinary tract infections: incidence, morbidity, and economic costs. *Am. J. Med.* 2002; 113 Suppl. 1A: 5S-13S.

[2] Ikaheimo, R., Siitonen, A., Heiskanen, T., et al. Recurrence of urinary tract infection in a primary care setting: analysis of a 1-year follow-up of 179 women. *Clin. Infect. Dis.* 1996; 22: 91-9.

[3] Hooton, T. M. Recurrent urinary tract infection in women. *Int. J. Antimicrob. Agents* 2001; 17: 259-68.

[4] Hickling, D. R., Nitti, V. W. Management of Recurrent Urinary Tract Infections in Healthy Adult Women. *Rev. Urol.* 2013; 15: 41-8.

[5] Albert, X., Huertas, I., Pereiro, I. I., et al. Antibiotics for preventing recurrent urinary tract infection in non-pregnant women. *Cochrane Database Syst. Rev.* 2004: CD001209.

[6] Harding, G. K., Buckwold, F. J., Marrie, T. J., et al. Prophylaxis of recurrent urinary tract infection in female patients. Efficacy of low-dose, thrice-weekly therapy with trimethoprim-sulfamethoxazole. *JAMA* 1979; 242: 1975-7.

[7] Lichtenberger, P., Hooton, T. M. Antimicrobial prophylaxis in women with recurrent urinary tract infections. *Int. J. Antimicrob. Agents* 2011; 38 Suppl.: 36-41.

[8] Melekos, M. D., Asbach, H. W., Gerharz, E., et al. Post-intercourse versus daily ciprofloxacin prophylaxis for recurrent urinary tract infections in premenopausal women. *J. Urol.* 1997; 157: 935-9.

[9] Zhong, Y. H., Fang, Y., Zhou, J. Z., et al. Effectiveness and safety of patient initiated single-dose versus continuous low-dose antibiotic prophylaxis for recurrent urinary tract infections in postmenopausal women: a randomized controlled study. *J. Int. Med. Res.* 2011; 39: 2335-43.

[10] Shepherd, A. K., Pottinger, P. S. Management of urinary tract infections in the era of increasing antimicrobial resistance. *Med. Clin. North Am.* 2013; 97: 737-57, xii.

[11] Beerepoot, M. A., ter Riet, G., Nys, S., et al. Cranberries vs antibiotics to prevent urinary tract infections: a randomized double-blind non-inferiority trial in premenopausal women. *Arch. Intern. Med.* 2011; 171: 1270-8.

[12] Hosein, I. K., Hill, D. W., Jenkins, L. E., et al. Clinical significance of the emergence of bacterial resistance in the hospital environment. *J. Appl. Microbiol.* 2002; 92 Suppl.: 90S-7S.

[13] Cosgrove, S. E. The relationship between antimicrobial resistance and patient outcomes: mortality, length of hospital stay, and health care costs. *Clin. Infect. Dis.* 2006; 42 Suppl. 2: S82-9.

[14] Nicolle, L. E. Urinary tract infection: traditional pharmacologic therapies. *Dis. Mon.* 2003; 49: 111-28.

[15] Den Heijer, C. D., Donker, G. A., Maes, J., et al. Antibiotic susceptibility of unselected uropathogenic Escherichia coli from female Dutch general practice patients: a comparison of two surveys with a 5 year interval. *J. Antimicrob. Chemother.* 2010; 65: 2128-33.

[16] Kahlmeter, G., Eco.Sens. An international survey of the antimicrobial susceptibility of pathogens from uncomplicated urinary tract infections: the ECO.SENS Project. *J. Antimicrob. Chemother.* 2003; 51: 69-76.

[17] Naber, K. G., Schito, G., Botto, H., et al. Surveillance study in Europe and Brazil on clinical aspects and Antimicrobial Resistance Epidemiology in Females with Cystitis (ARESC): implications for empiric therapy. *Eur. Urol.* 2008; 54: 1164-75.

[18] Gupta, K., Hooton, T. M., Stamm, W. E. Increasing antimicrobial resistance and the management of uncomplicated community-acquired urinary tract infections. *Ann. Intern. Med.* 2001; 135: 41-50.

[19] Schito, G. C., Naber, K. G., Botto, H., et al. The ARESC study: an international survey on the antimicrobial resistance of pathogens involved in uncomplicated urinary tract infections. *Int. J. Antimicrob. Agents* 2009; 34: 407-13.

[20] Falagas, M. E., Vouloumanou, E. K., Togias, A. G., et al. Fosfomycin versus other antibiotics for the treatment of cystitis: a meta-analysis of randomized controlled trials. *J. Antimicrob. Chemother.* 2010; 65: 1862-77.

[21] Falagas, M. E., Kastoris, A. C., Kapaskelis, A. M., et al. Fosfomycin for the treatment of multidrug-resistant, including extended-spectrum beta-lactamase producing, Enterobacteriaceae infections: a systematic review. *Lancet Infect. Dis.* 2010; 10: 43-50.

[22] Vellinga, A., Cormican, M., Hanahoe, B., et al. Predictive value of antimicrobial susceptibility from previous urinary tract infection in the treatment of re-infection. *Br. J. Gen. Pract.* 2010; 60: 511-3.

[23] Beerepoot, M. A., den Heijer, C. D., Penders, J., et al. Predictive value of Escherichia coli susceptibility in strains causing asymptomatic bacteriuria for women with recurrent symptomatic urinary tract infections receiving prophylaxis. *Clin. Microbiol. Infect.* 2012; 18: E84-90.

[24] Beerepoot, M. A., Geerlings, S. E., van Haarst, E. P., et al. Nonantibiotic Prophylaxis for Recurrent Urinary Tract Infections: A Systematic Review and Meta-Analysis of Randomized Controlled Trials. *J. Urol.* 2013.

[25] Hooton, T. M. Pathogenesis of urinary tract infections: an update. *J. Antimicrob. Chemother.* 2000; 46 Suppl. 1: 1-7; discussion 63-5.

[26] Moura, A., Nicolau, A., Hooton, T., et al. Antibiotherapy and pathogenesis of uncomplicated UTI: difficult relationships. *J. Appl. Microbiol.* 2009; 106: 1779-91.

[27] Jepson, R. G., Williams, G., Craig, J. C. Cranberries for preventing urinary tract infections. *Cochrane Database Syst. Rev.* 2012; 10: CD00 1321.

[28] Guay, D. R. Cranberry and urinary tract infections. *Drugs* 2009; 69: 775-807.

[29] Kontiokari, T., Sundqvist, K., Nuutinen, M., et al. Randomised trial of cranberry-lingonberry juice and Lactobacillus GG drink for the prevention of urinary tract infections in women. *BMJ* 2001; 322: 1571.

[30] Sengupta, K., Alluri, K., Golakoti, T., et al. A randomized, double blind,controlled, dose dependent clinical trial to evaluate the efficacy of a proanthocyanidin standardized whole cranberry (Vaccinium macrocarpon) powder on infections of the urinary tract. *Current Bioactive Compounds* 2011; 739–46.

[31] Stothers, L. A randomized trial to evaluate effectiveness and cost effectiveness of naturopathic cranberry products as prophylaxis against urinary tract infection in women. *Can. J. Urol.* 2002; 9: 1558-62.

[32] Barbosa-Cesnik, C., Brown, M. B., Buxton, M., et al. Cranberry juice fails to prevent recurrent urinary tract infection: results from a randomized placebo-controlled trial. *Clin. Infect. Dis.* 2011; 52: 23-30.

[33] Stapleton, A. E., Au-Yeung, M., Hooton, T. M., et al. Randomized, placebo-controlled phase 2 trial of a Lactobacillus crispatus probiotic

given intravaginally for prevention of recurrent urinary tract infection. *Clin. Infect. Dis.* 2011; 52: 1212-7.

[34] Falagas, M. E., Betsi, G. I., Tokas, T., et al. Probiotics for prevention of recurrent urinary tract infections in women: a review of the evidence from microbiological and clinical studies. *Drugs* 2006; 66: 1253-61.

[35] Beerepoot, M. A., ter Riet, G., Nys, S., et al. Lactobacilli vs antibiotics to prevent urinary tract infections: a randomized, double-blind, noninferiority trial in postmenopausal women. *Arch. Intern. Med.* 2012; 172: 704-12.

[36] Reid, G., Bruce, A., Taylor, M. Instillation of Lactobacillus and stimulation of indigenous organisms to prevent recurrence of urinary tract infections. *Microecol. Ther.* 1995; 23: 32-45.

[37] Barrons, R., Tassone, D. Use of Lactobacillus probiotics for bacterial genitourinary infections in women: a review. *Clin. Ther.* 2008; 30: 453-68.

[38] Raz, R. Postmenopausal women with recurrent UTI. *Int. J. Antimicrob. Agents* 2001; 17: 269-71.

[39] Luthje, P., Brauner, H., Ramos, N. L., et al. Estrogen supports urothelial defense mechanisms. *Sci. Transl. Med.* 2013; 5: 190ra80.

[40] Perrotta, C., Aznar, M., Mejia, R., et al. Oestrogens for preventing recurrent urinary tract infection in postmenopausal women. *Cochrane Database Syst. Rev.* 2008: CD005131.

[41] Raz, R., Stamm, W. E. A controlled trial of intravaginal estriol in postmenopausal women with recurrent urinary tract infections. *N. Engl. J. Med.* 1993; 329: 753-6.

[42] Eriksen, B. A randomized, open, parallel-group study on the preventive effect of an estradiol-releasing vaginal ring (Estring) on recurrent urinary tract infections in postmenopausal women. *Am. J. Obstet. Gynecol.* 1999; 180: 1072-9.

[43] Andersson, P., Engberg, I., Lidin-Janson, G., et al. Persistence of Escherichia coli bacteriuria is not determined by bacterial adherence. *Infect. Immun.* 1991; 59: 2915-21.

[44] Darouiche, R. O., Riosa, S., Hull, R. A. Comparison of Escherichia coli strains as agents for bacterial interference. *Infect. Control Hosp. Epidemiol.* 2010; 31: 659-61.

[45] Lutay, N., Ambite, I., Gronberg Hernandez, J., et al. Bacterial control of host gene expression through RNA polymerase II. *J. Clin. Invest.* 2013; 123: 2366-79.

[46] Sunden, F., Hakansson, L., Ljunggren, E., et al. Escherichia coli 83972 bacteriuria protects against recurrent lower urinary tract infections in patients with incomplete bladder emptying. *J. Urol.* 2010; 184: 179-85.

[47] Watts, R. E., Tan, C. K., Ulett, G. C., et al. Escherichia coli 83972 expressing a P fimbriae oligosaccharide receptor mimic impairs adhesion of uropathogenic E. coli. *J. Infect. Dis.* 2012; 206: 1242-9.

[48] Brumbaugh, A. R., Mobley, H. L. Preventing urinary tract infection: progress toward an effective Escherichia coli vaccine. *Expert Rev. Vaccines* 2012; 11: 663-76.

[49] Lorenzo-Gomez, M. F., Padilla-Fernandez, B., Garcia-Criado, F. J., et al. Evaluation of a therapeutic vaccine for the prevention of recurrent urinary tract infections versus prophylactic treatment with antibiotics. *Int. Urogynecol. J.* 2013; 24: 127-34.

[50] Asadi Karam, M. R., Oloomi, M., Mahdavi, M., et al. Vaccination with recombinant FimH fused with flagellin enhances cellular and humoral immunity against urinary tract infection in mice. *Vaccine* 2013; 31: 1210-6.

[51] Garenaux, A., Caza, M., Dozois, C. M. The Ins and Outs of siderophore mediated iron uptake by extra-intestinal pathogenic Escherichia coli. *Vet. Microbiol.* 2011; 153: 89-98.

[52] Garcia, E. C., Brumbaugh, A. R., Mobley, H. L. Redundancy and specificity of Escherichia coli iron acquisition systems during urinary tract infection. *Infect. Immun.* 2011; 79: 1225-35.

In: Urinary Tract Infections
Editor: Kristen E. Murrell
ISBN: 978-1-63117-180-2

Chapter 2

Urinary Tract Infections in Children: Epidemiology, Pathogenesis and Prevention

***Sonia Guadalupe Martínez Mejía*[1], *Martín Castillo de Vera*[2] *and Fermín García-Muñoz Rodrigo*[3]**

[1] Department of Pediatrics, Complejo Hospitalario Universitario Insular Materno-Infantil de Las Palmas de Gran Canaria, Spain

[2] General Pediatrics. Primary Health Care, Las Palmas de Gran Canaria, Canary Health Service, Spain

[3] Director of Neonatal Unit. Department of Pediatrics, Complejo Hospitalario Universitario Insular Materno-Infantil de Las Palmas de Gran Canaria, Spain

Abstract

Urinary tract infections (UTI) are among the most common bacterial infections in childhood. Its general incidence varies according to age and gender, but it is difficult to establish accurately because of the heterogeneity in UTI's definition, the population included, and the studies design and methodology.

In addition, symptoms in young children are frequently nonspecific. Some studies have shown a higher incidence of UTI in males than females during the first months of life, but this relation is reversed thereafter.

The estimated incidence in girls varies from 2.1% to 11.3%, and in boys from 1.0% to 3.6%, depending on age. As for the race, the available data suggests that the incidence of UTI is lower in African Americans as compared to White, Hispanic and Asian children.

The prevalence of acute pyelonephritis (APN) defined clinically (fever > 38.5°C, and C reactive protein > 20 mg/L) in pediatric patients with UTI is around 59% in boys and 32% in girls. Some studies using renal scintigraphy (DMSA) found a prevalence of APN in children with febrile UTI of 50-80%, while renal parenchymal inflammation was rarely found in lower tract infections. Although uncommon in children, renal abscesses are potential serious complications of UTI, but their incidence is also imprecisely known.

The most frequent pathogen involved in ascending infections is Escherichia coli, but Staphylococcus aureus is common after hematogenous dissemination. Acute focal bacterial nephritis is also rare in infancy although it could be an under-diagnosed condition.

The prevalence of vesicoureteral reflux (VUR) in the general population is around 1-3%, but in pediatric patients with UTI it ranges from 18% to 38%, and it is bilateral in half of the cases. Other nephro-urological structural anomalies that may contribute to the UTI pathogenesis are hydronephrosis and renal system duplication, present in 2.5-7.5% and 6-7% of cases, respectively.

The main etiological agent in childhood's UTI is Escherichia coli (70-90%). However, other bacteria should also be considered in children previously exposed to antibiotics, and among those hospitalized or with nephro-urological anomalies.

The infection usually starts with the perianal colonization by intestinal bacteria, with posterior invasion of the urethra, and ascending progression to other areas of the nephro-urological system.

While individual and genetic predisposition to UTI are recognized, the main factor favoring bacterial colonization and its progression to the upper urinary tract is the ability of the microorganisms to adhere to uroepithelial cells by pili or fimbriae (mainly the type 2 or P). This mechanism is favored by urinary stasis secondary to VUR and by obstructive processes that allow bacterial replication.

Given that bad voiding habits (infrequent emptying) and constipation are associated with an increased incidence of UTI, its correction, together with an increase in fluid intake may be beneficial to prevent bacterial multiplication and their migration to the upper urinary tract regions. Antibiotic prophylaxis should be considered in children with severe VUR (grades IV and V), genitourinary anomalies and recurrent infections. High-risk boys may also benefit from circumcision.

Introduction

Urinary tract infections (UTI) involve the presence of diverse microorganisms along the urinary tract. Therefore, the infection can affect anywhere from the urethra to the renal parenchyma, associating a variety of clinical symptoms and signs, and resulting in a lower UTI or an acute pyelonephritis/upper UTI.

UTIs represent one of the most frequent bacterial infections in childhood; it is estimated that 8% of girls and 2% of boys suffer an UTI before 16 years old, [1, 2] and that 30 to 50% of these children will suffer at least one recurrence. [3] Less frequently, UTIs can be produced by viruses and fungi. In these cases, special patient groups are usually affected.

To know the epidemiology of UTIs is essential to facilitate the evaluation of children with suspected UTI, since there are various subgroups with increased incidence and risk. Especially in infants and children between 2 months and 2 years old, UTIs often present with nonspecific symptomatology or with fever as the only symptom, and the risk of a UTI going unnoticed and the child suffering an occult bacteraemia is high. In addition to this difficulty, urine specimens for culture require invasive methods for collection (urethral catheterization or suprapubic aspiration), which delays diagnosis and treatment and increases the risk of developing an acute pyelonephritis. For these reasons, there are specific diagnostic and therapeutic guidelines for this age group.

In older children, the clinical symptomatology is more specific, with the presence of fever, flank or lower back pain, and urinary incontinence and dysuria, making diagnosis easier than for young children, because there are no problems with obtaining urine samples.

In contrast to children with fever or other symptomatology suggestive of a UTI, differentiating children with asymptomatic bacteriuria is important. In these children, finding of positive urine cultures is not accompanied by clinical symptoms. They have a normal physical examination and normal image studies. In these cases, antibiotic treatment is not indicated.

Most children with UTI recover soon and do not have any long-term complications, but a small subgroup is at risk of significant morbidity. This group of children falls into two categories: 1) those in which UTI may be the first sign of a serious underlying congenital anomaly—such as obstruction—that, if not relieved, will lead to more serious illness and also to renal damage; 2) those in which infections may be associated with progressive loss of kidney function, either in association with renal dysplasia, or with recurrent episodes of acute pyelonephritis/upper UTI. Therefore, it is important to develop clinical pathways to identify this small but important subgroup of children from the many children who present with infections and will recover without residual complications. [2]

The immediate objective of an appropriate diagnosis is to initiate antibiotic treatment to reduce the risk for renal scarring secondary to acute pyelonephritis, and to prevent long-term consequences, such as end-stage renal disease and hypertension, which is reported in approximately 5% of children with antecedent of recurrent UTI and/or related with vesicoureteral reflux (VUR). However, the long-term influence of these factors on future kidney function has been questioned in recent years, and we are seeing a trend toward less aggressive treatments and imaging studies of patients with UTI, giving special importance to prenatal ultrasound as the initial examination. [3]

Epidemiology

The incidence of UTI is difficult to estimate because the heterogeneity of epidemiological studies, including the definition of UTI, the variability of populations studied, and the methodology of sample collection. The total prevalence in febrile children younger than 2 years who are brought to the emergency departments is estimated to be nearly 7% (95% CI: 5.5–8.4%), and in children over 2 years with urinary symptomatology and/or fever, is estimated at nearly 7.8% percent (95% CI: 6.6–8.9%). [4] Chen et al. found a prevalence of 14% (95% CI: 11–17%) among febrile infants aged 1 to 24 months attending a pediatric emergency department, which is higher than in other studies. [5]

According to the NICE guidelines, data regarding incidence reveals that 2.1% of girls and 2.2% of boys will have had a UTI before the age of 2 years, and around 1/10 girls and 1/30 boys will have had a UTI by the age of 16 years. [2]

The case of neonates deserves special consideration, because UTI in this age differs from UTI in infants and children in several aspects: higher prevalence, greater incidence in male sex, higher frequency of infections produced by bacteria different to *Escherichia coli*, and higher risk of urosepsis. [6] In a multicenter prospective study in febrile neonates and infants younger than 60 days, Zorc et al. found an overall risk for UTI of 9%. [7] Kanellopoulus et al., in a retrospective study to evaluate the first episode of UTI in neonates and infants, observed higher incidence in male newborns than in females, but a similar distribution by sex after the neonatal period.[8]

In the cases of infants with unexplained fever, it is important to identify groups at high risk for UTI, to seek laboratory confirmation and, when indicated, to establish appropriate antibiotic treatment to avoid clinical deterioration and long-term renal damage. In addition to age, other non-modifiable factors such as sex, circumcision state, race, and sexual activity, can influence UTI development; [4, 9] awareness of different prevalence rates in each group helps the physician to estimate the likelihood of UTI in a given patient. Other factors to consider are the presence of structural or functional urinary anomalies and previous UTI episodes, which significantly increase the probability of UTI.

For febrile children between 2 months and 2 years old, the risk of UTI is greater especially in cases of unexplained fever higher than 39ºC and that lasts for more than 48 hours, and if the patient has a previous history of UTI, he is an uncircumcised male, and presents with a *diseased appearance* and suprapubic tenderness. [10] Consideration to the role of age on the increased risk of UTI justifies the existence of clinical guidelines focused on diagnosis and treatment of UTI in this age group.

The prevalence of UTI in children older than 2 years and adolescents is variable, and in adolescents, one must consider sexual intercourse as one of the most relevant risk factors, mainly in girls, to develop acute cystitis.

Studies that investigate the relationship between UTI, gender, and age, found a greater prevalence among male patients during the first 3 months of life, which declined thereafter. Among female patients, prevalence rates are higher during the first 12 months of life. [4] A study by Hiraoka et al. of patients with febrile UTI showed that 73% of them had their first UTI before the age of 7 months, and that was more frequent in boys (94%), than girls (37%). [11]

A study, performed by Ginsburg et al., in hospitalized patients with UTI (mean age 2.1 months) found that under 3 months of age 75% of cases corresponded to boys and 25% to girls. Between 3 and 8 months, 11% were male and 89% female patients. [12]

Several studies have found an increased risk of UTI in uncircumcised boys. In a meta-analysis by Shaikh et al. [4] the prevalence of UTI in circumcised boys was 2.4% (CI: 1.4% – 3.5%), and in uncircumcised 20.1% (CI: 16.8% – 23.4%). In this study the prevalence of UTI among febrile uncircumcised infants younger than 3 months of age was 20.1%. [4] For this reason circumcision seems to be a protective factor against UTI, but the risk-benefit of this intervention remains still unclear.

Heterogeneity exists among studies with regard to the influence of race. Data seem to indicate that in developed countries, the prevalence of UTI is higher in white children. Shaikh et al. observed that the prevalence of UTI was significantly higher in white (8%; CI: 5.1% – 11.0%) than in African American children (4.7%; CI: 2.1% – 7.3%). [4] In the same way, Chen et al. observed a higher prevalence of UTIs in Asian (22%), followed by white (16%) and Hispanic children (16%), with African American children showing the lowest prevalence (4%). [13] It has been suggested the possibility that the blood group may be a protective factor against the attachment of bacteria to the uroepithelium, but this issue is far from been clear. [13]

Other factors may influence prevalence of UTI: febrile status, genitourinary anomalies, VUR, sexual activity, use of urinary catheter, bladder dysfunction or neurogenic bladder. All of them must be taken into consideration when caring for a patient with a possible UTI, to assess their individual risk.

To accurately know the rates of UTI recurrence in children is difficult. An estimated 30 – 50% will have at least one recurrence. [3] The risk of recurrence is considered higher in girls, and they usually experience more episodes than boys. Children who present early in life with a UTI are more prone to recurrent infections: three-quarters of children presenting before the age of 1 year will have a recurrence. After this age, approximately 40% of girls and 30% of boys will have a recurrence. Girls, but not boys, have increasing rates of recurrence with age. These findings appear to be related to reported age-specific prevalence data on asymptomatic bacteriuria. [2]

Etiopathogenia

Microbiology

Bacteria are the main cause of urinary tract infection. *E. coli* is the most common bacterial cause of UTI, accounting for 70–90% of cases. [14, 15, 16] Previous exposure to antibiotics, history of hospitalization, younger age, and urological anomalies or instrumentation increase the likelihood of other etiologic agents such as Proteus mirabilis, Klebsiella spp. and Pseudomonas aeruginosa. [16, 17] Other less common microorganisms that may cause UTI include *Enterobacter cloacae, Citrobacter spp., Serratia marcescens, Morganella morganii,* or *Acinetobacter spp.* Possible etiologic gram-positive bacteria include *Staphylococcus saprophyticus*, *Enterococcus faecalis*, and rarely *Streptococcus agalactiae and Staphylococcus* aureus. [16]

The presence of *P. mirabilis* is usually found in uncircumcised boys older than 1 year, and is associated with renal calculi. In cases of UTI produced by *S. aureus*, other sites of infection via hematogenous spread, renal abscess, and pyelonephritis should be considered. *E. coli* and *S. saprophyticus* are the principal pathogenic agents in UTI of sexually active females. [18]

Viruses and fungi are uncommon causes of UTI. Implicated viruses include adenoviruses, enteroviruses, coxsackie viruses, BK poliomaviruses, and echoviruses, which generally produce lower UTI, with hemorrhagic cystitis by adenovirus being the most common. [17, 18]

Fungal UTIs are associated with immunosuppression, preterm neonates, long-term use of broad-spectrum antibiotic therapy, and indwelling urinary catheter. The main causative fungi are *Candida spp, Aspergillus spp, and Cryptococcus* neoformans. [19]

In neonates, *E. coli* is also the most common causative pathogen (77.4% of cases), followed by *group B Streptococcus*. *E. coli* is more frequent in community-acquired UTI (83.2%) than in nosocomial UTI (49%), which are mainly caused by *Klebsiella pneumoniae, Enterobacter spp., Enterococcus spp., Pseudomonas spp., and Candida spp.* [6, 12] The latter of these is more frequent in preterm neonates, representing 42% of cases. [20]

Pathogenesis

The pathogenesis of UTI is usually based on *E. coli* models. The causative bacteria generally originate in the gastrointestinal tract, and the principal mechanism to produce UTI is ascendant. Bacterial flora in the periurethral area acts as a defensive barrier. The first step to produce a UTI is the alteration of this flora and colonization of the periurethral area by enteric pathogens.

In newborns, the prevalence of upper urinary tract infections, the existence of urinary tract abnormalities, and the association between UTI and bacteremia are all greater than in older children. [6] Magin et al. in a retrospective study found that 12.4% of blood cultures from neonates admitted for UTI were positive. [21]

The importance of the ascending mechanism is well recognized, but the haematogenous spread as origin of UTI in newborns is questioned, although it should be considered in case of bacteremia and when *S. aureus* is the causative agent. [12, 22]

The localization and severity of UTI depends on the magnitude of the immune response resulting from the bacteria-host interaction. The principal host factors are the age, sex, genetic factors, ethnicity, constipation, bladder dysfunction (for example, in spina bifida), lack of circumcision, sexual activity, existence of VUR, or bladder catheterization.

Urgency and voiding dysfunction constitute the principal cause of UTI in schoolgirls, and usually, the diagnosis of UTI is delayed because symptoms may go unnoticed for parents. Also, routine anamnesis may ignore this issue, making UTI a frequently under-diagnosed problem. Urgency and voiding dysfunction appears in 8.4% of girls and 1.7% of boys of school age with a history of recurrent UTI, and these are functional entities that usually occur at jointly. In voiding urgency, detrusor hyperactivity exists without involvement of the pelvic musculature. This is contrary to dysfunctional urination with hyperactivity of the latter. [23] Frequently, children with voiding dysfunction present VUR, and its persistence increases the risk for upper UTIs and renal scarring.

The bacterial factors include the presence of P. fimbriae, or "pili" in some *E. coli*, which allow adherence to the uroepithelium and ascent to the kidney, [24] and *P. mirabilis'* ability to produce and secrete urease, which causes alkalinization of urine pH and promotes the formation of bacteria-containing staghorn calculi to allow self-perpetuating infection. [25]

Approximately 10% to 15% of pyelonephritis cases can produce renal scarring and loss of renal parenchyma. The development of renal scarring has been associated with: recurrent febrile UTI, delay in treatment of acute infection, virulence of uropathogens, bowel and bladder dysfunction, obstructive malformations, and VUR at early ages. [26, 27] When this damage is unilateral and focal (the most frequently observed) the remaining renal tissue hypertrophies to maintain the renal function. Damaged areas that are multiple, bilateral, or on a unique kidney, may produce progressive loss of renal function.

Prevention

After a first symptomatic UTI episode, up to one-third of infants and 30% to 50% of older children are prone to recurrence, and this susceptibility is highest within the 2 to 6 months following initial infection. [3, 6]

In general, preventive measures aimed to decrease recurrences of UTI should be individualized. The pattern of urinary tract dysfunction or the urinary bad habits of the patient should be taken into account. An important objective is to achieve an appropriate liquid intake by the patient. [15]

Hygienic Measures

In boys and girls with UTI and/or signs of lower urinary tract dysfunction, investigating and treating the presence of constipation is recommended to prevent recurrence of UTI. [2, 15] Given that bad voiding habits (infrequent emptying) and constipation are associated with an increased incidence of UTI, its correction, together with an increase in fluid intake, may be beneficial to prevent bacterial multiplication and migration to the upper urinary tract regions, especially in school age children. In girls with urgency and dysfunctional urination, symptoms may also be accompanied by vaginal discharge. Treatment and prevention include education of children and parents, avoiding constipation, adoption of hygienic measures, such as separating the legs during urination for the free-flow of the urine stream in girls, or seated urination for boys; maintaining a voiding diary, including the frequency and volume of urination; ensuring frequent urination (every 3 hours); and maintaining a generous liquid intake. Children who have had a UTI should have ready access to clean toilets when required and should not be expected or forced to delay voiding.[2] These measures usually simultaneously correct voiding dysfunction and low-grade VUR. For infants and children younger than 2 years, who are not toilet-trained, it is important to insist on adequate genital hygiene and prevention of stool retention.

Antibiotic Prophylaxis

The use of antibiotic prophylaxis has greatly changed in the last few years, becoming more restrictive, and is no longer routinely recommended in infants and children following first UTI, though it may be considered in infants and children with recurrent UTI. Asymptomatic bacteriuria in infants and children should not be treated with prophylactic antibiotics. [2, 15, 28] Antibiotic prophylaxis has been used to reduce the risk of recurrent, symptomatic UTIs and the subsequent development of renal scarring and parenchymal defect. Prophylaxis is believed to prevent or decrease acute symptomatic UTI and to prevent the development of new renal scarring in children with or without VUR. Consequently, its use implicates the additional need to assess the urinary tract for VUR and renal parenchymal defects in healthy children after recovery from the acute episode.

Several recent studies have discredited this belief about the beneficial use of antibiotic prophylaxis, which must be balanced against potential risks.

Chronic antibiotic use has several disadvantages for the individual and for the population as a whole, including hepatotoxicity, gastrointestinal, and hematologic disorders, the emergence of bacterial resistance, etc. [3]

In a recent study conducted to assess the role of prophylactic antibiotics, Craig et al., observed that long-term prophylaxis with low-dose trimethoprim–sulfamethoxazole was associated with a modest decrease in the number of symptomatic UTIs in predisposed children, with a reduction in the absolute risk of 6%, meaning that 14 children would need to be treated to prevent one case of recurrent UTI. The pattern of recurrence suggested that the benefit of antibiotic therapy was greatest during the first 6 months of treatment, the most likely time for recurrent infection, concluding that any benefits of long-term antibiotic use in reducing the risk of new kidney damage from pyelonephritis remain speculative. [29] All this evidence questions the effectiveness of long-term low-dose prophylaxis in the prevention of recurrent symptomatic UTIs or progressive renal scarring.

In summary, for children with recurrent UTI, it is recommended to evaluate the indication for antibiotic prophylaxis individually, after a complete study to rule out structural or functional anomalies of the urinary tract, taking into account the existence of resistant strains. Current indications for antibiotic prophylaxis in some centers include high-grade (III–V) VUR and urinary tract anomalies involving dilation with obstruction. Antibiotic prophylaxis is recommended for girls with VUR grades III–V, and for boys with VUR grades IV–V, during one year or until control assessment of VUR grade with voiding cystourethrogram. [15]

In infants and children presenting with urinary tract dilatation and suspected obstruction, antibiotic prophylaxis has been recommended until confirmation of diagnosis and obstruction treatment. Most recent studies in this group of patients have shown a low incidence of UTI. Roth et al. detected an incidence about 4.3% in untreated patients with antenatal diagnosed upper urinary tract obstruction (hydronephrosis grades 3 or 4) during a median follow-up period of 2 years. [30] Mami et al. followed 2 month-old infants with isolated moderate renal pelvis dilatation (anterior to posterior diameter of 10 to 15 mm) over 12–14 months and found a similar rate of UTI in the patient group as in an age-matched control group, suggesting that antibiotic prophy laxis should not be administered in those cases. In a group of infants with severe dilatation (>15 mm or equal to 20 mm), the incidence of UTI was significantly higher than in a control group (13.9% vs. 2.5%), suggesting the necessity of careful observation, but not initiation of prophylaxis. [31] However, obstructive megaureters significantly increased the risk of pyelonephritis, with a mean of 1.3 UTI episodes per patient, and an incidence reduction of 55% during the first year of life after receiving antibiotic prophylaxis. [32]

Circumcision

Although circumcision is known to reduce the risk of UTI during the first year of life, routine circumcision should not be recommended. The main role of this procedure is in boys with a history of recurrent UTI, complex structural urinary anomalies, or high-grade VUR, because the benefits in these cases may outweigh the risk of complications. [2] The number of circumcisions needed to prevent one UTI is estimated to be nearly 111 in the general population, 11 in boys with recurrent UTI, and 4 in the case of boys with high-grade VUR. [33] These data show that circumcision may be a little cost-effective strategy for the general population, and that should be better reserved for boys at high risk of UTI and renal damage. [3, 34] Some guidelines recommend for these risk groups—before circumcision—medical treatment with topical steroid, which causes retraction of the foreskin in about 60% of the treated patients. [6]

Other Preventive Strategies

Current strategies include behavior modification, which does not imply costly interventions. Other strategies include regular intake of cranberry juice or reduced intake of caffeinated and high-sugar drinks. However, it does not exists enough scientific evidence to support other recommendations such as uropathogenic strain vaccines, ascorbic acid, cranberry juice, or probiotics.[2] The use of cranberry products has increased in the last few years. Its proposed mechanism of action is the inhibition of *E. coli* adhesion to the uroepithelium lining of the bladder wall. One of the potential problems in demonstrating effectiveness of cranberry products is that the active ingredient (proantho-cyanidin) is only effective for approximately 10–12 h; therefore, to be effective, a patient would need to consume two glasses a day for an indefinite period of time. Furthermore, cranberry juice is calorific and sweet, is likely to be expensive, and some people find it unpalatable, with side effects such as gastrointestinal discomfort. At this time, tablets and capsules should not be recommended unless they clearly contain the recommended amount of proanthocyanidin—at least 36 mg/day. Salo et al. conducted a randomized trial on 263 children with UTIs to receive either cranberry juice or placebo for 6 months and followed them for one year, and found that the intervention did not significantly reduce the incidence of recurrent UTI. [35, 36]

The use of probiotics to prevent UTI is being explored. Probiotics act by displacing pathogenic bacteria from the gut and boosting innate immunity. Several studies suggest that these effects may help to prevent and eliminate the colonization of pathogenic bacteria in the gut, and that such a reduction in the fecal load of uropathogens will translate to a reduction in the incidence of recurrent UTI. The few studies conducted in children, however, have found no differences in UTI incidence while using cranberry juice or placebo. [2, 15]

References

[1] Feld L, Mattoo T. Urinary tract infections and vesicoureteral reflux in infants and children. *Pediatrics in Review*. 2010;31;451-63.

[2] National Collaborating Centre for Women's and Children's Health. Commissioned by the National Institute for Health and Clinical Excellence (NICE). Urinary Tract Infection in Children: *diagnosis, treatment and long-term management*. 2007.

[3] Paintsil E. Uptodate on recent guidelines for the management of unariry tract infections in children: the shifting paradigm. *Curr. Opin. Pediatr.* 2013;25:88-94.

[4] Shaikh N, Morone NE, Bost JE, Farrell MH. Prevalence of urinary tract infection in childhood: a meta-analysis. *Pediatr. Infect. Dis. J.* 2008;27:302–8.

[5] Chen L, Baker MD. Racial and Ethnic Differences in the Rates of Urinary Tract Infections in Febrile Infants in the Emergency Department. *Pediatr. Emerg Care*. 2006;22:485-7.

[6] Beetz R. Evaluation and management of urinary tract infections in the neonate. *Curr. Opin. Pediatr.* 2012;24:205-11.

[7] Zorc JJ, Levine DA, Platt SL, et al. Clinical and demographic factors associated with urinary tract infection in young febrile infants. *Pediatrics* 2005; 116:644–48

[8] Kanellopoulos TA, Salakos C, Spiliopoulou I, et al. First urinary tract infection in neonates, infants and young children: a comparative study. *Pediatr. Nephrol*. 2006;21:1131-7.

[9] Hooton TM, Scholes D, Hughes JP, et al. A prospective study of risk factors for symptomatic urinary tract infection in young women. *N. Engl. J. Med*. 1996;335:468-74.

[10] Shaikh N, Morone NE, Lopez J, et al. Does this child have a urinary tract infection? *JAMA*. 2007;298:2895-904.

[11] Hiraoka M, Tsukahara H, Ohshima Y, Mayumi M. Meatus tightly covered by the prepuce is associated with urinary infection. *Pediatr. Int.* 2002;44:658-62.

[12] Ginsburg CM, McCracken GH, Jr. Urinary tract infections in young infants. *Pediatrics*. 1982;69(4):409-12.

[13] Chen L, Baker M. Racial and ethnic differences in the rates of urinary tract infections in febrile infants in the emergency department. Pediatr *Emerg. Care.* 2006;22(7):485-7.

[14] Capdevila Cogul E, Martín Ibáñez I., Mainou Cid C, Toral Rodríguez E, Cols Roig M, Agut Quijano T, Caritg Bosch J. and Camarasa Piqué F. First-time urinary tract infection in healthy infants: epidemiology, diagnosis and treatment. *An. Esp. Pediatr.* 2001; 55: 310-14.

[15] Working Group of the Clinical Practice Guideline on Urinary Tract Infection in the Pediatric Population. Clinical Guideline on Urinary Tract Infection in the Pediatric Population. Quality Plan for the National Health System. Ministry of Health, Social Policy and Equality. Aragon Institute of Health Sciences; 2011. Clinical Practice Guidelines, in the NHS: I + CS No 2009/01.

[16] Eiros Bouza J, Ochoa Sangrador C. Grupo Investigador del Proyecto. Etiological profile of urinary tract infections and antimicrobial susceptibility of urinary pathogens. *An. Pediatr.* (Barc). 2007;67:461-8.

[17] Friedman S, Reif S, Assia A, Mishaal R, Levy I. Clinical and laboratory characteristics of non-E. coli urinary tract infections. *Arch. Dis. Child.* 2006;91:845-6.

[18] Feld L, Mattoo TK. Urinary Tract Infections and Vesicoureteral Reflux in Infants and Children. *Pediatrics in Review*. 2010; 31: 451-63.

[19] Sobel JD, Vazquez JA. Fungal infections of the urinary tract. *World J. Urol.* 1999;17:410-4.

[20] Phillips JR, Karlowicz MG. Prevalence of Candida species in hospital-acquired urinary tract infections in a neonatal intensive care unit. *Pediatr Infect. Dis. J.* 1997;16(2):190.

[21] Magin EC, Garcia-Garcia JJ, Sert SZ, et al. Efficacy of short-term intravenous antibiotic in neonates with urinary tract infection. *Pediatr Emerg. Care*. 2007; 23:83–6.

[22] Littlewood JM. 66 infants with urinary tract infection in first month of life. *Arch. Dis. Child.* 1972;47:218-26.

[23] Lucio Delgado A., Ariceta Iraola G., Oliver Linares F., Blanco Bruned J. Recurrent urinary infections: "It s not reflux, it s the bladder". *An. Pediatr. (Barc).* 2010;72:231-3.

[24] Honkinen O, Lehtonen OP, Ruuskanen O, et al. Cohort study of bacterial species causing urinary tract infection and urinary tract abnormalities in children. *BMJ.* 1999;318:770-1.

[25] Mobley HL, Island MD, Massad G. Virulence determinants of uropathogenic Escherichia coli and Proteus mirabilis. *Kidney Int. Suppl.* 1994;47:S129-36.

[26] Lin KY, Chiu NT, Chen MJ, et al. Acute pyelonephritis and sequelae of renal scar in pediatric first febrile urinary tract infection. *Pediatr. Nephrol.* 2003;18:362-5.

[27] Ataei N, Madani A, Habibi R, Khorasani M. Evaluation of acute pyelonephritis with DMSA scans in children presenting after the age of 5 years. *Pediatr. Nephrol.* 2005;20:1439-44.

[28] Subcommittee on Urinary Tract Infection, Steering Committee on Quality Guideline for the Diagnosis and Management of the Initial UTI in Febrile Infants and Children 2 to 24 Months. *Pediatrics.* 2011; 128,595-611.

[29] Craig et al., Investigators for the Prevention of Recurrent Urinary Tract Infection in Children with Vesicoureteric Reflux and Normal Renal Tracts (PRIVENT). Antibiotic prophylaxis and recurrent urinary tract infection in children. *N. Engl. J. Med.* 2009;361:1748-59.

[30] Roth CC, Hubanks JM, Bright BC, et al. Occurrence of urinary tract infection in children with significant upper urinary tract obstruction. *Urology* 2009; 73:74–78.

[31] Mami C, Paolata A, Palmara A, et al. Outcome and management of isolated moderate renal pelvis dilatation detected at postnatal screening. *Pediatr. Nephrol.* 2009;24:2005–8.

[32] Islek A, Guven AG, Koyun M, et al. Probability of urinary tract infection in infants with ureteropelvic junction obstruction: is anti-bacterial prophylaxis really needed? *Pediatr. Nephrol.* 2011;26: 1837–41.

[33] Singh-Grewal D, Macdessi J, Craig J. Circumcision for the prevention of urinary tract infection in boys: a systematic review of randomised trials and observational Studies. *Arch. Dis. Child.* 2005;90:853–8.

[34] American Academy of Pediatrics Task Force on Circumcision. Male circumcision. *Pediatrics* 2012; 130:e756–e785.

[35] Jepson RG, Williams G, Craig JC. Cranberries for preventing urinary tract infections (Review). The Cochrane Library 2012. Cochrane Database Syst Rev. 2012 Oct 17;10:CD001321. doi: 10.1002 /14651858. CD001321.pub5.

[36] Jepson R, Webster A. Cranberries for preventing urinary tract infections. Cochrane Commentaries. *Nephrology*. 2013.18:388–9.

In: Urinary Tract Infections
Editor: Kristen E. Murrell

ISBN: 978-1-63117-180-2

Chapter 3

Virulence Factors of Uropathogenic *Escherichia coli* and Their Role in Development of Urinary Tract Infection

Tara Vollmerhausen and Mohammad Katouli**[*]**
Inflammation and Healing Research Cluster, School of Health and Sport Sciences, Faculty of Science, Health, Education and Engineering, University of the Sunshine Coast, Maroochydore DC, Australia

Abstract

Uropathogenic *Escherichia coli* (UPEC) are the major etiological agent of urinary tract infections (UTIs). UPEC differ from non-pathogenic *E. coli* by the presence of virulence factors which enable these bacteria to colonize uroepithelial cells and to establish a UTI. These include a range of adherence factors, toxins, iron uptake systems, and capsules. Evolutionary influences on the acquisition and main role of virulence genes amongst *E. coli* are widely debated, with some research holding that the prevalence of strains with virulence genes increases the likelihood of infection, whereas other believe that virulence genes provide a selective advantage for infection of extraintestinal sites. UPEC strains causing UTI are often found among the faecal flora of the host.

[*] Corresponding author: A/ Prof Mohammad Katouli. Email: mkatouli@usc.edu.au.

The presence and persistence of these strains in the gastrointestinal (GI) tract is facilitated by their adhesion to intestinal epithelial cells. This may serve as a source for the development of UTI if their numbers increases and dominate the *E. coli* population of the GI tract in the host.

Introduction

E. coli is a commensal inhabitant of the large intestine of humans that colonizes the gastrointestinal (GI) tract of infants within hours of birth [1-3]. Although a majority of *E. coli* strains live in the gastrointestinal (GI) tract without causing infection, some have acquired the ability to cause life-threatening intestinal or extraintestinal infections such as Cholera-like diarrheal disease, urinary tract infection (UTI), meningitis and sepsis [4]. *E. coli* strains that cause UTI are known as uropathogenic *E. coli* or UPEC. The pathogenesis of UPEC is a multi-step process attributable to the acquisition of virulence genes, with factors involved in adhesion, colonization and survival in the urinary tract [3]. Bacteria that colonize the urinary tract ascend towards the bladder to cause cystitis, which is associated with the classic symptoms of a UTI such as pain, frequency, and urgency. Some *E. coli* are able to migrate from the GI tract to colonize the vaginal introitus and periurethral area before ascending the urethra to cause infection [5-9]. UPEC possess a collection of virulence factors that enhance their ability to survive the hostile environment of the urinary tract. Many of these virulence factors are involved in adhesion and survival of UPEC in the GI tract, which is considered a primary reservoir of UPEC. Thus factors that promote intestinal colonization may be of significance in the pathogenesis of UTI. This chapter reviews the importance of virulence factors of UPEC and their role in the migration of *E. coli* from the GI tract to urinary tract.

Colonization of the Colon and Vagina

Colonization of the Colon

Bacteria that enter the GI tract encounter various digestive enzymes secreted by the intestines. In addition, these bacteria also face the gut-associated lymphoid tissue (GALT), intestinal mucus and lysozyme secretions, which aid in decreasing bacterial adhesion to intestinal epithelial cells [10].

Mucous can trap bacteria and prevent them from adhering to epithelial cells [11]. GALT helps to prevent bacterial adhesion via secretory IgA (sIgA) which is initially secreted by lymphocytes of the lamina propria as IgA and transferred into the mucus layer through a secretary component of the gut epithelial cells [12]. SIgA binds with the adhesive organelle type 1 fimbriae to trap *E. coli* in mucous and to prevent their adhesion [13]. The lower GI tract has a high rate of cell turnover, constantly shedding epithelial cells as well as bacteria which have been able to adhere to them. These host defences help to prevent and decrease bacterial adhesion and colonization in the lower GI tract [11].

The primary habitat of *E. coli* is the large intestine of humans. Before birth the GI tract is sterile, however after birth *E. coli* is often the first bacterium to colonize the intestine of infants [14]. Several factors including the mode of delivery [15], diet [16] and low birth weight [17] can influence bacterial species that colonize the intestines of infants. In the GI tract, *E. coli* must compete with other bacteria for nutrients and space, and need to penetrate the mucous layer to colonize the mucosa. It has been suggested that *E. coli* predominantly digests gluconate, a sugar found in mucous, which enables them to occupy this highly specific metabolic niche to become part of the resident flora [3, 18]. Few studies have focused on the habitat and selective pressures on commensal strains in the GI tract, and the impact they have on adhesion of potentially pathogenic *E. coli*. The relationship between humans and *E. coli* is generally regarded as commensalism, whereby the host provides nutrients, a stable environment, transportation, and dissemination [18]. In exchange, indigenous microflora provide colonization resistance to potential pathogens by occupying available adhesion sites along the GI tract, preventing their adhesion and colonization to cause infection [18].

Most strains persist in the GI tract without causing infection. *E. coli* that are able to persist become part of the resident microflora. In contrast to transient strains that stay in the GI tract for a short period of time, usually days to weeks, the resident strains can be found for up to months or years and normally dominate the *E. coli* population of the gut as they adhere and colonize the epithelial cell of the GI tract [6, 19]. The ability for *E. coli* to colonize the GI tract is an important first step in causing UTI. Whilst microflora of the GI tract remains relatively stable, factors such as diet and antibiotic treatment have been shown to destabilize the microflora, which can lead to decreased colonization resistance and overgrowth of certain bacteria. Moreno et al. (2008) found 30 out of 42 patients experiencing cystitis carried the *E. coli* capable of causing UTI as the dominant faecal strains. These findings reinforce the importance of gut as a major reservoir for UTI-causing strains. Little is known about the factors that lead to an increase in the number of UPEC in the GI tract of patients with UTI, however research has eluded to include dietary changes, increased emotional stress, and antibiotic treatment [5]. Resident strains display characteristics that facilitate their persistence in the GI tract including adhesive molecules, capsules and iron acquisition systems [6, 20]. Interestingly the same virulence factors enhance survival of *E. coli* in the hostile environment of the urinary tract. However, UPEC possess virulence genes that distinguish them from other commensal *E. coli*, encoding for factors that allow attachment to the uroepithelium, to help avoid host detection and to scavenge for nutrients in the urinary tract [21].

Colonization of the Vagina

Colonization of the vaginal introitus with *E. coli* originating from the GI tract often precedes episodes of UTI and can serve as a constant reservoir in close proximity for bacteria to enter the bladder [22]. Vaginal strains of *E. coli* have been shown to share common virulence gene profiles and serotypes with UPEC isolated from cases of UTI, further supporting the notion that the vagina can provide a reservoir of UPEC for transmission to the bladder [9]. *E. coli* have been identified as part of the vaginal microflora in 9 – 28% of non-pregnant women, and in 24 – 31% of pregnant women [9]. Among pregnant women, vaginal colonization of *E. coli* is associated with low birth weight in infants [23], and an increased risk of neonatal septicaemia and meningitis [24]. Women with recurrent UTI more often have abnormal flora of the urogenital tract when compared to healthy women [25]. Stamey and co-workers demonstrated that among premenopausal women without a history of UTI, *E. coli* only transiently colonized the vaginal introitus [26]. However, the establishment of dominant clones of UPEC in the vaginal introitus often immediately preceded a recurrent UTI [26].

Vaginal microflora is largely influenced by estrogen, which leads to increased glycogen in vaginal epithelial cells, and its metabolism further lowers vaginal pH leading to the selection of acid-tolerant bacteria such as lactobacilli [27]. Disruption of the resident vaginal microflora, such as in postmenopausal women who frequently experience decreased vaginal estrogen and pH, can facilitate the colonization of UPEC. This is supported by studies that found postmenopausal women who frequently experience UTI, were more likely to harbor *Enterobacteriaceae* in the vaginal introital [28].

The microenvironment of the vaginal introitus is quite distinct to that of the urinary tract. The bladder and kidneys are composed of a transitional and cuboidal epithelium, respectively [29]. In contrast, the vaginal mucosa is composed of a squamous epithelium with a hierarchy of differentiated cell layers [30]. Although the receptors for type 1 fimbriae in the urinary tract are well defined, less is known about vaginal receptors. *E. coli* have been shown to have increased adherence to vaginal epithelial cells isolated from women susceptible to recurrent UTI compared to cells obtained from healthy controls [31]. Differentiation of vaginal epithelial cells has been shown to increase the surface expression of mannosylated proteins, promoting type 1 fimbriae mediated adherence [30]. The fact that some women are more prone to recurrent UTI may be associated with differential glycoprotein processing which regulates mannosylated proteins on vaginal epithelial cells [30].

Migration to the Periurethral Region

The tissue surrounding the urethra is known as the periurethral region. Intermittent colonization of the periurethral tissue can function as a platform for the transmission of UPEC to the urinary tract. The presence of certain aerobes and anaerobes as part of the urethral flora in women of reproductive age is considered a host defence mechanism [32]. There is evidence to suggest that normal flora is able to inhibit the growth of other species, such as *Bacteroides melaninogenicus* inhibiting the growth of aerobic Gram-negative rods [33]. A study on the urethral flora of women of different ages found no aerobic Gram-negative bacilli in women of reproductive age, however half of postmenopausal women included in the study contained these bacteria [32]. Changes in normal urethral flora among postmenopausal women may contribute to increased susceptibility to recurrent UTI amongst this group.

Risk Factors Associated with UTI

Risk factors associated with UTI can be considered behavioural or non-behavioural. A number of studies have reported that sexual intercourse is associated with UTI among young women [34, 35]. Sexual intercourse can facilitate the movement of UPEC from the introitus to the bladder. Diaphragm and spermicide use has also been associated with UTI [34, 36]. Spermicide nonoxynol-9 has been shown to enhance the adherence of *E. coli* to vaginal epithelial cells, and to exhibit a greater bactericidal effect towards normal vaginal organisms [37]. Together, the use of spermicide provides a selective advantage for *E. coli* within the vagina, increasing the number of UPEC colonising the vagina.

A number of host risk factors have been identified. Common risk factors include previous incidences of UTI and a family history of UTI [35]. Many women with a history of recurrent UTI have underlying host factors that predispose them to infection. Women who are not secretors of blood group antigens have an increased risk of developing recurrent UTIs [38]. Non-secretor women selectively expressed sialosyl galactosyl globoside (SGG) and disialosyl galactosyl globoside (DSGG) on uroepithelial and vaginal epithelial cells [39]. SGG is the receptor for the major uropathogenic adhesin, P-fimbriae, involved in binding to the kidney during pyelonephritis [40]. Therefore it is not surprising that non-secretor status among women is associated with pyelonephritis [41]. The presence of SGG plays an important role to increase binding of UPEC to uroepithelial and vaginal epithelial cells [40].

Behavioural factors do not play as big of a role in UTI in women after menopause [42]. Estrogen deficiency associated with menopause is considered to increase a woman's risk to a range of diseases including UTI [43]. For instance, it has been shown that the rate of recurrent UTIs increases to 53% among women who are at least 55 years old [44]. Estrogens plays an important role in modulation of the mucosal barrier [45]. Postmenopausal hormonal changes in women have been shown to be associated with disruption of the normal vagina microflora, decreasing the presence of lactobacilli and enhancing colonization of *E. coli* which subsequently increases the chance of migration of these bacteria to the bladder. Estrogen therapy among postmenopausal women has been shown to reduce recurrent UTIs [46]. Recently, vaginal estrogen supplementation was shown to enhance lower urinary tract mucosal defences among postmenopausal women [47]. This study found that the expression of genes encoding antimicrobial peptides and tight junctions were lower among postmenopausal women, as compared with premenopausal women, but their expression was induced by vaginal estrogen supplementation [47]. Clinical data indicates that vaginal estrogen delivery is more effective than oral estrogen replacement therapy in preventing recurrent UTIs in postmenopausal women [42].

Hostile Environment of the Urinary Tract

Among women, the opening of the urinary tract is in frequent contact with bacteria due to close proximity to the vagina and GI tract. Despite the constant presence of bacteria, the incidences of UTIs are less frequent. This may raise the question that what keeps the urinary system healthy? Some of the most important protective mechanisms of the urinary tract are the regular emptying of the bladder and the flushing effect of the urine that washes bacteria as well as the valve mechanisms [48].

The bladder has to withstand frequent changes in urine volume with constant stretching and contracting of the epithelial cells. The bladder mucosa is composed of transitional epithelial cells and is lined with highly differentiated and multinuclear superficial facet or umbrella cells [29]. The apical side of these umbrella cells contain integral membrane proteins known as uroplakins, which are a receptor for the common UPEC-associated adhesin type 1 fimbriae [29]. The basal side of umbrella cells consists of intermediate and basal cells, and beneath the basement membrane is the lamina propria [29]. The role of the urinary tract is to drain liquids and excrete urine from the body, therefore bladder epithelial cells are often exposed to cytotoxic substances, varying pH levels, and changes of osmolality [48]. Despite these constant changes, UPEC survive quite well in urine.

Low availability of nutrients, especially of iron, is a common feature of the urinary tract. Upon detection of an infection an immune response known as hypoferremia further reduces iron availability to bacteria [49, 50] by decreasing iron absorption from the GI tract and storing it intracellularly [51]. Furthermore, the release of transferrin from host cells tightly binds free iron, limiting the availability of iron for bacteria [52, 53]. When bacteria first enter the urinary tract they come into contact with the uroepithelium and encounter lactoferrin, another iron binding host compound. The recruitment of neutrophils to the site of infection leads to increased secretion of lactoferrin from secondary granules [54].

Lactoferrin also exhibits antibacterial activity, binding to LPS of bacterial walls to affect membrane permeability leading to cell lysis [55]. This combination of factors makes the urinary tract a hostile environment for bacterial survival.

Virulence Factors of UPEC

UPEC possess a range of virulence genes that enable their survival and infection in the urinary tract [56]. It has been shown that pathogenesis of UPEC is a multi-step process, with virulence factors involved in adhesion, colonization, invasion, survival, and damage to the host [3]. Many of these virulence factors are controlled by phase-variable genetic switches that are dependent on environmental conditions [21, 57], allowing differential expression of certain virulence factors as *E. coli* move from the GI tract to colonize the bladder. Table 1 summarises factors involved pathogenesis of UPEC.

Table 1. Virulence factors and characteristics of UPEC that enable them to colonize the urinary tract and establish infection

Virulence Factor	Feature	Role in pathogenesis
Adhesin	Type 1, P, DR, S and curli fimbriae	Adhesion to mucosal epithelium
Flagellum	H antigens	Facilitates motility and ascension from the bladder to kidneys
Host defense avoidance	Capsular polysaccharides, LPS, serum resistance, outer membrane proteins	Evasion of immune recognition
Exported virulence factors	CNF1, α-hemolysin	Toxins can alter host signaling and lead to host cell death

Fimbriae-mediated adherence is important for virulence of UPEC. Bacterial attachment in the urinary tract is central to establishing an infection. In this process, the presence of adhesin molecules is arguably the most important determinant of pathogenicity. UPEC must be able to adhere to uroepithelial cells of the urinary tract to avoid rapid clearance with the flow of urine. Common adhesins associated with UPEC include type 1 fimbriae, P-fimbriae, S/F1C family of fimbriae and the DR family of adhesins [21]. The role of these adhesins in pathogenesis of UPEC is briefly discussed below.

Type 1 Fimbriae

Receptors and Epidemiology of Type 1 Fimbriae

Type 1 fimbriae are highly prevalent filamentous organelles that facilitate attachment to epithelial surfaces [58, 59]. These fimbriae are encoded by the *fim* gene cluster, composed of structural components encoded by *fim*A, *fim*F, *fim*G, and *fim*H, and pilus components *fim*C and *fim*D [60]. Type 1 fimbriae are expressed by more than 90% of both pathogenic and commensal *E. coli* strains [58]. Although the prevalence of the adhesive tip, FimH, does not indicate any correlation with uropathogenic strains [21], its expression is crucial to mediate binding to urethral epithelial cells during the initial stages of infection [61, 62]. The FimH adhesin at the tip of type 1 fimbriae recognizes D-mannose moieties on cell-bound and secreted glycoproteins [63, 64], and has also been shown to facilitate mannose-sensitive binding to nonglycosylated peptide epitopes [65]. Uroplakin 1a serves as the uroepithelial receptor for type 1 fimbriae [66]. Type 1 fimbriae have also been shown to adhere to intestinal [67] and vaginal cells [68] and probably help residency of UPEC in GI tract. Interestingly, postmenopausal women have been shown to have a lower expression of uroplakin 1a in uroepithelial cells, which can be restored by vaginal estrogen therapy [47].

Role of Type 1 Fimbriae in the Urinary Tract

Host defenses at the epithelial cell barrier can prevent bacterial attachment by the production of Tamm-Horsfall protein (THP) [69]. A major role of THP is to prevent bacterial colonization by binding with type 1 fimbriae to inhibit fimbrial interaction with uroplakin receptors [70, 71]. (172,193). THP is an abundant protein in urine which is produced in the thick ascending limb of the loop of Henle [72]. THP coats the surface of uroepithelial cells to bind to type 1 fimbriae and prevent UPEC adherence. Evidence suggests that THP may also have an important role in the regulation of the innate and adaptive immunity of the urinary tract [73].

Attachment by type 1 fimbriae allows bacteria to gain a foothold in the urinary tract to avoid being swept away during micturition. UPEC have intuitively used this defense mechanism to their advantage. Through the formation of catch-bonds upon FimH binding to mannose moieties, type 1 fimbriae adherence is actually strengthened by the sheer stress induced by the flow of urine [74]. Type 1 fimbriae also have an important role mediating invasion of host cells for the formation of intracellular bacterial communities [75]. The ability of UPEC to invade the uroepithelium contributes to the persistence and recurrence of UTIs [76, 77]. Once attached, UPEC can enter epithelial cells by membrane-bound vacuoles [78]. Type 1-piliated *E. coli* can mediate host cell invasion through the recognition of integrins [59]. The adhesive tip of type 1 fimbriae, FimH, binds to α3 and β1 integrin on uroepithelial cells, initiating signaling cascades which stimulate the host plasma membrane to zipper around and encase attached UPEC [59]. Once internalized, UPEC exist in membrane bound-acidic compartments [77]. UPEC that enter facet cells can then go on to multiply rapidly and form intracellular bacterial communities [79].

After UPEC have adhered, the host can initiate a cascade of responses to clear a bacterial infection, some of which are trigger by binding of type 1 fimbriae. An important host mechanism during UTIs is the ability of infected bladder epithelial cells to be exfoliated [80]. Type 1 fimbriated bacteria induce apoptosis, which is a process of programmed cell death [59]. Epithelial exfoliation appears within hours of initial adhesion, helping to clear adhered UPEC from an early stage [81]. Exfoliation and the influx of immune cells can damage the uroepithelium and potentially expose deeper underlying tissue layers where bacteria can gain access to form quiescent intracellular reservoirs (QIRs) [59, 82, 83]. QIRs can persist latently for months before potentially serving a seeds to cause recurrent infections. Invasion of epithelial cells allows bacteria to colonize, multiply, and to exist transiently as intracellular bacterial communities [84]. Type 1 fimbriae also plays an important role to activate the host inflammatory response by the recognition of type 1 fimbriae by mast cells, leading to the typical symptoms associated with UTI [85].

Many extraintestinal *E. coli* possess mutations in the binding tip of type 1 fimbriae, FimH, providing an advantage in colonization of extraintestinal sites [30, 86]. Naturally occurring amino acid replacements in FimH increase the monomannose-binding capacity of FimH [87-89]. These differential binding abilities of FimH have been observed among pathogenic and commensal strains, with 80% of *E. coli* isolates from human intestines expressing low-binding to mannose, as opposed to 70% of *E. coli* causing UTI showing high-binding to mannose [87]. These high-binding mutations are more common among UPEC than commensal *E. coli.* Although type 1 fimbriae is prevalent amongst commensal and pathogenic *E. coli*, allelic variations of FimH are likely to favor survival in extraintestinal sites.

Role of Type 1 Fimbriae in the GI Tract

As discussed previously, the GI tract constitutes an important reservoir for UPEC that follow the faecal-vaginal-urethral route, for which the presence of virulence genes is believed to enhance their migration and survival. Type 1 fimbriae bind to mannose-containing glycoproteins on epithelial cells of the small and large intestines [90]. They can also bind to the mannose-containing sIgA present in intestinal mucus [64]. Although there is a high prevalence of type 1 fimbriae amongst faecal isolates [91], the role these fimbriae play in intestinal colonization remains uncertain [67, 92, 93]. A study using HeLa cells found type 1 fimbriae did not contribute to the ability of *E. coli* to colonize the large intestine [6]. In further support of these results, no difference in the prevalence of type 1 fimbriae was observed between resident and transient *E. coli* clones of the GI tract [6]. Other researchers have suggested these fimbriae bind to colonic cells and substances loosely associated with the epithelium [94]. Among the protective defences of the GI tract is sIgA, which is secreted in mucous and has been shown to bind mannose containing oligosaccharide to aggregate bacteria and prevent their adherence to GI epithelial cells [13]. Binding of sIgA to type 1 fimbriae to trap *E. coli* in mucous on the other hand helps commensal *E. coli* to produce a biofilm in the GI tract which further prevents pathogenic bacteria from adhering to epithelial cells [13].

P-Fimbriae

Receptors and Epidemiology of P-Fimbriae

Pyelonephritis-associated pili, or P-fimbriae, are the second most common adhesin amongst UPEC [21]. These fimbriae are more important for colonization of the upper urinary tract, with up to 80% of pyelonephritis strains expressing P-fimbriae [93, 95-97]. P-fimbriae are assembled by a family of proteins that form the *pap* gene cluster. Of these, PapG is the tip of the pilus responsible for adhesion to epithelial cells [21]. Genes encoding P-fimbriae (*pap* genes) are located on the chromosome and the cluster is composed of a major subunits *pap*A, genes involved in the adhesin tip *pap*E, *pap*F and *pap*G, processing and regulatory genes *pap*C, *pap*D and *pap*H, and the regulatory genes *pap*B and *pap*I. The expression of *pap* genes varies in response to temperature, glucose and amino acid concentrations. P-fimbriae bind to the α-D-galactopyranosyl-(1-4)-β-D-galactopyranoside (Galα(1-4)Gal moiety) which occur in the series of P-blood group antigen-specific glycosphingolipids [98-100]. These renal glycolipids are abundant in epithelial cells lining the upper urinary tract.

The Role of P-Fimbriae in the Urinary Tract

P-fimbriae are recognised as a key determinant in the virulence of UPEC to mediate attachment to tissues of the kidney. A review by Johnson 1991 identified 70% of *E. coli* causing pyelonephritis expressed P-fimbriae compared to 36% of cystitis isolates [21]. P-fimbriae facilitate binding to epithelial cells by the PapG adhesin positioned at the distal end of the fibrillum [101-103]. PapG mediates binding to the receptor Galα(1-4)Gal or the globo series of glycolipids in the human kidney [104]. There are three variations of the PapG tip with slightly different binding ability and include PapG allele I, PapG allele II, and PapG allele III [101-103]. The prevalence of PapG allele I is uncommon [102], however it has been observed amongst uropathogenic isolates in some studies [105]. PapG allele II is associated with pyelonephritis [106] whereas cystitis is associated with PapG allele III [107].

After mediating adherence to uroepithelial cells, P-fimbriae play an additional role to establish a robust inflammatory response in the kidney, which in turn leads to kidney damage during pyelonephritis [106, 108]. Attachment of P-fimbriae to renal epithelial cells activates the ceramide-signalling pathway which further contributes to the induction of cytokines [109]. The release of ceramide activates Toll-like receptor 4 signalling and elicits an immune response [110]. This immune response contributes to the production of interleukin (IL)-6, IL-8 and an influx of neutrophils to the site [111]. Furthermore, P-fimbriated *E. coli* have been shown to resist the bactericidal actions of neutrophils [112]. P fimbriae have been shown to elicit an adaptive response to ensure their survival in the kidney through the suppression a key local immune defence, sIgA [113].

The Role of P-Fimbriae in the GI Tract

Although P-fimbriae are established virulence factors of *E. coli* causing extraintestinal infections, their role in intestinal colonization is not well defined. Intestinal epithelial cells have been shown to express receptors for P-fimbriae [67]. Resident *E. coli* strains of healthy adults have been shown to express P-fimbriae, suggesting a role for their attachment to the intestinal epithelium and intestinal colonization [92]. Persistence of UPEC in the GI tract has been suggested to be associated with the class II allele of P-fimbriae [20, 114].

A review by Johnson 1991 reported that 52% of all urinary *E. coli* expressed P-fimbriae compared to 19% of faecal isolates [21]. The binding of P-fimbriae to Gal-Gal receptors is stronger to the urinary epithelium than that to colonic epithelial cells, suggesting that the P-fimbriae organelle has been tailored for adherence in the urinary tract [115]. It has been shown that Gal α(1-4) Gal-containing receptors are located in surface-associated substances as opposed to in the cell membrane of colonic cells [64, 67]. Furthermore, continuous shedding of colonic epithelial cells containing Gal-Gal receptors could form an ecological niche for commensal *E. coli* to establish colonization within the intestinal tract [64]. Nonetheless, it appears that P-fimbriae mediated colonization of the GI epithelium is an important first step in the migration of UPEC to the urinary tract to cause infection.

S Family of Fimbriae

S fimbriae were firstly discovered among *E. coli* causing pyelonephritis as a group of fimbriae that bound to sialic acid containing structures, sialyl galactosides [116]. The adhesive tip of S fimbriae, the major subunit SfaS, interacts with sialic acid residues located on uroplakin III of kidney epithelia cells including vascular endothelial cells of the kidney [80, 117]. In addition to SfaS, minor subunit SfaA can also mediate binding [118]. The abundance of uroplakin III on the lumenal surface of the bladder suggests that S fimbriae have an important role in cystitis. S fimbriae have also been shown to contribute to nephropathogenicity by mediating attachment to eukaryotic cells [119]. S fimbriae are often associated with ascending UTIs, sepsis, and meningitis [119, 120]. The gene encoding the major subunit SfaS has been identified in 14% of UPEC and 47% of neonatal meningitis *E. coli* [121]. The carriage of genes encoding S fimbriae has been identified in up to 20% of intestinal *E. coli* strains [20]. However, despite their presence in faecal isolates, S fimbriae are not associated with intestinal persistence, a factor which may be associated with sialic acid being present as a mucin molecule rather than facilitating attachment to epithelial cells [114].

Another member of the S family of fimbriae, i.e., F1C fimbriae, are encoded by the major subunit proteins FocA and minor subunits FocF and FocH [122]. F1C fimbriae are genetically homologous to S fimbriae, differing in receptor specificity [120, 123]. F1C fimbriae binds to the Gal NAcβ1-4Galβ sequence of glycolipids that are expressed on epithelial cells found in the distal tubules and collecting duct in the kidney and by bladder endothelial cells [124]. This fimbriae is expressed by approximately 14% of *E. coli* causing UTI and 7% of faecal isolates [125]. F1C fimbriae have been shown to be important for biofilm formation and contribute to murine intestinal colonization for the intestinal probiotic strain *E. coli* Nissle 1917 [126].

DR Family of Fimbrial Adhesins

The DR family of fimbriae is associated with *E. coli* causing ascending UTIs, especially pregnancy-associated pyelonephritis, and intestinal infections. *E. coli* with DR fimbriae are present in up to 30% patients with pyelonephritis, and is expressed in about half of *E. coli* isolated from children with cystitis [21, 127]. Patients with UTI caused by *E. coli* carrying DR fimbriae are twice as likely to experience a recurrent infection [128].

The DR family of fimbriae adhesins includes the DR adhesin and F1845, afimbrial adhesins AFA-I, AFA-II, AFA-III, AFA-IV, and non-fimbrial adhesins Nfa-I and DR-II [129]. The DR family of adhesins interact with the DR blood group antigen present on decay accelerating factor (DAF, also known as CD55) expressed on erythrocytes in the uroepithelium [129]. Receptors for DR are located in the intestines and the urinary tract, however DR hemagglutinin is not associated with intestinal persistence [114]. The gene encoding the DR-binding adhesins, *afa/dra*BC, has been identified in 5% of faecal *E. coli* [130]. The increased expression of DAF receptors during pregnancy is believed to be a factor associated with increased incidence of pyelonephritis during this period [131]. Binding of the DR family of adhesins can trigger signal transduction pathways which results in the activation of phosphatidylinositol 3-kinase (PI-3-kinase) and expression of the major histocompatibility complex (MHC) molecule MICA [3, 132]. The cytopathic effect of the DR family is characterized by long cellular extensions from host cells that envelop UPEC [3, 133].

Autotransporters

A further group of adhesins is represented by the autotransporter proteins. Antigen 43 (Ag43) is a well characterized autotransporter involved in persistence of *E. coli* in the urinary tract. Ag43 has been identified in up to 79% of *E. coli* causing UTI, and is associated with persistent or relapse UTI, indicating that it plays an important role for recurrent UTI [134]. We have observed a higher prevalence of the gene encoding Ag43 in *E. coli* causing UTI among hospitalized adults compared to children (unpublished data). Ag43 is a self-recognizing surface protein that causes autoaggregation by an intercellular handshake mechanism [135]. Expression of Ag43 is co-regulated with the production of type 1 fimbriae, with the latter being phenotypically dominant to Ag43 [135]. The production of type 1 fimbriae creates a physical barrier that prevents self-recognition of Ag43 and the handshake mechanism [135]. Expression of type 1 fimbriae and Ag43 are phase variable, allowing bacteria to sequentially colonize tissue in the urinary tract [136]. Ag43 is regulated by OxyR, which is involved in the response to oxidative stress. OxyR-mediated regulation of Ag43 and expression of biofilm formation may protect *E. coli* from prolonged exposure to oxidative stress [136]. Ag43 is expressed on the surface of *E. coli* in intracellular bacterial communities [79], and has been shown to promote long-term persistence in the urinary tract in mice [137].

Bacterial Biofilm Formation

It is commonly accepted that bacteria often exist in nature as part of a bacterial matrix irreversibly attached to a surface known as a biofilm [138, 139]. Biofilms are widespread and can be found in water, soil, and in the human body. Biofilms in the human body are common on the skin, in the mouth and in the GI tract. They are also found on medical devices such as urinary catheters, making bacteria more resistant to antibiotic treatment and difficult to eradicate. Additionally, in the human host, bacteria existing as part of a biofilm are less susceptible to the host immune response [140]. Bacteria living in a biofilm function differently to planktonic bacteria, exhibiting coordinated multicellular behavior with a decreased growth rate. Exopolysaccharides are an important component in biofilms and can protect bacteria against harmful substances such as oxidizing agents and antibiotics

[140, 141]. To establish a biofilm, bacteria must first adhere to a surface. Initially bacterial adhesion is reversible however, the production of exopolymeric substances leads to irreversible attachment. Once firmly attached, bacteria then replicate and develop into a fully mature biofilm, after which single motile bacteria are able to disperse to infect new sites. The bacterial environment as part of a biofilm is different to that experienced by planktonic cells, that is, they experience high cell density, and oxygen and nutrient limitations. Furthermore, gene expression amongst bacteria existing as part of a biofilm is different from that of planktonic bacteria, with up to 38% of the *E. coli* genome expression affected during biofilm formation [142-144]. The lifestyle change from planktonic to sessile is a well-coordinated and complex process involving many genes. Of major importance during biofilm formation are the genes involved in the adhesion of bacteria to physical surfaces, mediated by the expression of extracellular structures. Bacterial biofilms are composed of a matrix of proteins, deoxyribonucleic acid (DNA), ribonucleic acid (RNA), and polysaccharide polymers [145]. Common polysaccharide polymers include β-1,6-*N*-acetyl-D-glucosamine polymer (PGA), colonic acid, and cellulose [146, 147]. Biofilm formation has been shown to be mediated by type 1 fimbriae, Antigen 43 (Ag43), flagella, curli fimbriae and cellulose [136, 146, 148, 149].

Curli Fimbriae and Cellulose

Bacterial attachment is promoted by another structure known as curli fimbriae. Curli are thin proteinaceous fimbriae that enhance bacterial cell-cell aggregation [150, 151]. Curli bind to host proteins fibronectin and plasminogen [152, 153], and promote invasion of eukaryotic cells [154]. Curli expression during extraintestinal infections is associated with an increased induction of pro-inflammatory cytokines [155, 156].

Whilst many bacteria carry the genes coding for curli, this fimbriae is not expressed in many laboratory *E. coli* strains due to CsgD promoter silencing [157]. Curli production is organized from two divergently transcribed operons *csg*BA and *csg*DEFG. The *csg*BA operon encodes *csg*A which is the major subunit for curli fimbriae. The *csg*DEFG operon contains the regulatory gene *csg*D which influences regulation of curli formation. Curli are often co-expressed with another CsgD regulated component known as cellulose. Co-production of cellulose and curli results in a strong and rigid hydrophobic extracellular matrix [147]. Curli and cellulose synthesis are common amongst clinical *E. coli*, suggesting an important role in host-pathogen interactions [155, 156].

Cellulose is a highly hydrophilic polysaccharide consisting of a chain of β (1→4) linked D-glucose units with high mechanical strength [158]. Microbial cellulose provides an extracellular protective coating for bacteria that has been observed amongst a range of pathogenic and commensal bacteria [150, 156, 159]. Although cellulose has been shown to lead to the formation of a rigid biofilm at the air-liquid interface in some bacterial strains [144], cellulose production is not strictly correlated with biofilm formation [160], and in some instances cellulose can inhibit the formation of biofilm [161]. Cellulose production can also enhance biofilm formation by reducing motility [162]. Amongst pathogenic *E. coli*, cellulose co-expression with curli fimbriae has been shown to counteract curli-mediated adherence to epithelial cells [156, 163, 164]. Cellulose producing bacteria have been shown to induce a lower IL-8 response during infection and to persist longer in the urinary tract [156]. The ability to express cellulose was also found to be more pronounced in *E. coli* causing recurrent UTIs than strains cultured from sporadic UTIs, suggesting cellulose is an important bacterial factor for long-term persistence [165]. Cellulose aggregates have been shown to increase in low iron environments [166], further suggesting an important role for cellulose production in survival of UPEC in the iron limited urinary tract. Cellulose synthesis depends on the expression of two divergent operons, *bcs*ABZC and *bcs*EFG, which are constitutively transcribed [147, 167]. While BcsA and BcsB form the cellulose synthase complex, the operon also contains a cellulase gene BcsZ [168]. Although the function of cellulase in a cellulose synthase operon is not well understood, production has been speculated to allow bacteria to rapidly escape from a cellulose matrix in response to changes in environmental conditions [166].

Toxins of UPEC

Hemolysins

E. coli hemolysin is a calcium-activated pore-forming cytotoxin with specificity towards many host cells [169-171]. Hemolysin plays a major role in kidney damage during pyelonephritis by causing superoxide anion stimulation and hydrogen peroxide release from the host to damage tubular cells [172]. Hemolysin can also lead to inflammation, tissue damage, and disruption of phagocyte function [170, 173-175]. The toxin leads to the formation of membrane lesions which is further associated with an influx of calcium ions and an efflux of potassium ions [176]. Among erythrocytes, this leads to colloid-osmotic lysis. More recently, alpha-hemolysin has been shown to lead to rapid uroepithelial shedding and hemorrhage [177]. It has also been speculated that inhibition of cytokines by alpha-hemolysin early during infection allows UPEC to establish a niche prior to activation of the immune response [178]. Among *E. coli* causing human infections, alpha-hemolysin is encoded chromosomally by the gene *hly*A [179, 180]. Hemolysin production is regulated by iron availability with increased expression during times of low iron concentration [172, 181]. Hemolysin production is often associated with urinary and sepsis isolates, but is not common among commensal isolates [21, 182]. Among urinary isolates, hemolysin production is more common among E. coli stains from patients with pyelonephritis [21]. The production of a hemolysin is believed to contribute to chronic pyelonephritis amongst children [183]. The production of hemolysin and P-fimbriae has been shown to be the two most important factors in pathogenesis of UPEC [184, 185].

Cytotoxic Necrotising Factor

Cytotoxic necrotising factor 1 (CNF1) is another toxin of *E. coli* commonly expressed in up to 40% of UPEC [186]. CNF1 targets the Rho family of GTP-binding proteins, causing changes that include actin cytoskeleton reorganisation, multinucleation and cell spreading, and apoptosis of uroepithelial cells, which facilitates bacterial invasion into deeper tissue layers of the urinary tract [187, 188]. CNF1 is often co-expressed with other virulence factors in UPEC strains and is encoded chromosomally by the *cnf*1 gene [21, 189]. Haemolysin and CNF1 are associated with *E. coli* strains from patients with UTI rather than faecal isolates [190, 191].

Iron Siderophores

A common feature of the urinary tract is the low availability of nutrients, especially of iron. Iron is an important nutrient for the survival of UPEC. Therefore it is not surprising that UPEC change their gene expression in iron limited environments [192]. The ability of bacteria to obtain sufficient iron is linked with virulence. UPEC possess a range of mechanisms to overcome host defenses to facilitate iron acquisition from within the iron-limited environment of the urinary tract [53]. Within the human host iron is bound with proteins such as hemoglobin and heme [193] and the uptake of iron by bacteria is mainly through siderophores, small iron-chelating molecules, which bind to iron with high affinity [194]. Various studies have highlighted the importance of iron in *E. coli* pathogenesis, with increased expression of genes involved in iron and siderophore biosynthesis amongst *E. coli* isolated from the urine of mice compared to those grown in nutrient rich medium [192]. Siderophores function in different ways, some scavenge iron whilst others compete with the host to release iron from transferrin and lactoferrin [51, 53]. Iron is transported into the cell via outer membrane receptor proteins on the surface of the bacterium specific for each siderophore system [51]. Common uropathogenic siderophores include aerobactin, salmochelin, yersiniabactin, and enterobactin [194].

a) Aerobactin, a hydroxamate siderophore, is a bacterial iron chelating agent which helps *E. coli* to sequester iron in low-iron environments. It has been strongly associated with pyelonephritis, cystitis, and bacteremia as opposed to asymptomatic bacteriuria or faecal strains [21, 195]. Aerobactin is also associated with bacterial persistence in the GI tract, and is more common amongst resident than transient *E. coli* strains hence it may give a competitive advantage for long term survival [20, 115, 192]. In the host, the immunogenic aerobactin receptor is inactivated by a host protein tear lipocalin [196].
b) Enterobactin is a highly conserved catecholate siderophore of commensal and pathogenic *E. coli* that binds to Fe^{3+} with high affinity [197]. The role of enterobactin in virulence is unclear, with some studies finding enterobactin did not contribute to virulence [198]. Enterobactin has been shown to have a fundamental role in colonization of the murine intestinal tract [199]. In the host, enterobactin is inactivated by serum albumin and siderocalin, a host protein that inhibits bacterial iron acquisition by binding ferric catecholates [200]. Additionally, human neutrophil gelatinase-associated lipocalin (NGAL) can bind to ferric enterobactin with high affinity [196].
c) The salmochelin siderophore systems is encoded in the *iro*A locus [201]. The siderophore system salmochelin, a C-glucosylated enterobactin, with its catecholate receptor IroN not only functions as an iron uptake receptor, but also promotes bacterial cell invasion [202]. Additionally, the IroN receptor is involved in the transport of

the siderophore enterobactin [203], an ability that would enhance survival in a mixed community such as the GI tract, a major reservoir of UPEC. Catecholate siderophores are more important for colonization of the urinary tract compared to other types of siderophores [204]. Unlike enterobactin, salmochelin is not inactivated by lipocalin 2, a host protein which avidly binds catecholate siderophore enterobactin, representing a unique innate immune evasion strategy [205]. This catecholate siderophore is associated with pathogenesis of UPEC [24, 201].

d) The yersiniabactin siderophore system is encoded by the *irp* gene cluster with the receptor FyuA. Yersiniabactin is highly conserved in chromosomal DNA and is widely distributed amongst extraintestinal *E. coli* causing UTI and septicemia [206]. Expression of Yersiniabactin and salmochelin are correlated, suggesting that they may exhibit complementary activities [207]. FyuA is upregulated and is required for efficient biofilm formation in iron limited environ-ments [208]. Recently, yersiniabactin has been found to provide copper resistance, mediated by the ability to sequester host derived Cu(II), preventing its reduction to Cu(I) [209].

The presence of multiple siderophore systems among UPEC is thought to allow pathogens to take advantage of multiple iron sources during the course of infection as they move to new environments [210]. No virulence factor alone is enough for a strain to cause a UTI. Rather, a strain requires a complementary set of virulence factors that function together to enable a bacteria to interact with the environment and to colonize the urinary tract [211, 212]. Whilst defined pathotypes exist for enteric *E. coli*, a defined UPEC pathotype has not been established.

Capsule and Serum Resistance

A common characteristic of UPEC is the secretion of surface structures, such as O-antigens and K capsules, which act to protect the bacteria from the host immune system and to enhance survival of bacteria against the antimicrobial activities of serum [213, 214]. More than 80 distinct capsular polysaccharides, designated K antigens have been identified in *E. coli.* Capsules are made up of repeating carbohydrate subunits that coat the bacterium. This coating interferes with O-antigen detection, shielding the bacterium from phagocytosis. The capsules of most UPEC strains are group II polysaccharides, including K1 and K5. These capsules are often acidic and highly anionic, characteristics which act as a sponge to sequester and neutralize antimicrobial peptides [215]. Capsules also help to shield bacteria from phagocytosis by blocking activation of the alternative complement pathway. The capsule polysaccharide interferes with C3b binding, allowing the bacterium to evade opsonization, ingestion and destruction by phagocytes. Capsules have also been shown to influence biofilm formation by weakening initial cell surface contact and inhibiting biofilm maturation [216, 217].

Whilst capsule synthesis is common amongst faecal isolates, synthesis is more frequency associated with *E. coli* causing extraintestinal infections [218]. Capsule synthesis is common amongst *E. coli* causing invasive infections such as septicemia and meningitis [219]. Common K antigens among UPEC include K1, K5, K30 and K92 [21].The K1 capsule is the most common type among extraintestinal infections such as UTI, septicemia and meningitis [21]. *E. coli* expressing K1 capsule are the major cause of Gram-negative bacteremia and meningitis in neonates [220]. The production of K1 and K5 capsules are also common in resident strains of the GI tract [201, 221]. The K1 capsule is poorly immunogenic due to molecular mimicking of polysialic acid found on certain host cells [222]. K1 capsule has been revealed to contribute to intracellular bacterial communities formation, reducing neutrophil induction and enhancing generational replication when compared to a capsular mutant, however the function of capsular polysaccharide in IBC development remains unclear [223]. Not surprisingly, K1 strains are more likely to possess the virulence-associated adhesion, P fimbriae, than strains of other capsular types [224].

The ability for capsular polysaccharide to shield the bacterium from phagocytosis and the immune complement system is likely to increase survival in serum. Many invasive pathogens express polysaccharide capsules on their surfaces which protect them against immune defense mechanisms. Serum resistance is represented by the ability for a bacterium to resist killing by the complement system in the presence of serum. It is often linked with strains isolated from patients with more invasive infections such as pyelonephritis and cystitis than those from patients experiencing asymptomatic bacteriuria or from faecal strains [21]. Capsular polysaccharide and O-polysaccharide side chains of *E. coli* are believed to contribute to serum survival.

In *E. coli*, the outer membrane protein *tra*T mediates serum resistance via interference with complement-mediated killing [21]. Although *tra*T is common among extraintestinal *E. coli*, it is only associated with serum resistance among UPEC [225].

Serogroups and Serotypes

Serotyping of *E. coli* based on the somatic (O), flagellar (H) and capsular (K) polysaccharide antigens is commonly used in epidemiological studies. The O antigen is made up of repeating side chains of LPS, while the K antigen is composed of polysaccharides, and the H antigen is determined from the structure of flagellin [226]. The serogroup of a strain refers to its O antigen type, whereas its serotype refers to two or all three O, K and H antigens. A characteristic set of these antigens defines to which serotype a strain belongs, with UPEC often sharing the same O antigens or O:K serotypes. The association of certain serotypes with specific pathotypes provides useful information in clinical settings. Common uropathogenic serogroups include O1, O2, O4, O6, O7, O8, O16, O16/72, O18, O2, O50 and O75 [21]. Not surprisingly, virulence factors of UPEC are also associated with serogroups common in infection [227]. Traditionally, the method for serotyping is a laborious process involving the use of cross-absorbed antisera for 167 O antigens, 74 K antigens and 56 H antigens [228]. However, in the past decade alternative serogroup molecular methods have been developed to make serotyping faster and less laborious [229, 230].

Formation of Intracellular Bacterial Communities

Women have up to a 44% chance of a recurrent infection within 12 months of the UTI [44]. In up to 77% of cases, recurrent UTIs are caused by reinfection with the same *E. coli* responsible for the primary infection [8, 231, 232]. Recurrent infection with the same strains may be due to the ability of *E. coli* to invade bladder epithelium and mast cells to potentially protect themselves from the effects of antibiotics [75]. This has been demonstrated using a mouse model of UTI, and it has been suggested that *E. coli* can lie dormant within the bladder mucosa [76].

Once attached, *E. coli* can be internalized by epithelial cells into membrane-bound vacuoles [78]. The ability of UPEC to invade the uroepithelium contributes to the persistence and recurrence of UTIs [76, 77]. Invasion of epithelial cells allows UPEC to colonize, multiply, and persist as intracellular bacterial communities (IBCs) [84]. The discovery of intracellular biofilm-like pods in bladder epithelia of mice lacking an intact innate immune response suggested a new reservoir for the persistence of UPEC within the bladder [79]. These biofilm-like pods were later called IBCs. Many similarities have been noted between IBCs and biofilms, with the suggestion that bacteria in IBCs act the same as those forming biofilms on innate surfaces [233]. Once inside epithelial cells, bacteria grow in biofilm-like communities Hunstad and Justice 2010). Type 1-piliated *E. coli* can mediate host cell invasion through the recognition of integrins [59]. β1 integrin is expressed in epithelial cells of the urinary tract, making it a common receptor for uropathogens [59, 82]. It has previously been demonstrated that FimH is able to bind to β1 integrins, triggering cytoskeleton rearrangement to mediate entry into host cells [59]. The presence of β1 integrin throughout bladder superficial cells allows UPEC to enter superficial umbrella cells, which is often followed by programmed cell death and exfoliation [59, 82, 83]. Type 1 fimbriae, Ag43 and capsules are important to form aggregates within the host cell cytosol and subsequently to develop mature IBCs. Capsule may be required for the condensation of the IBC community [79, 234]. The importance of non-capsular polysaccharides, such as cellulose, in the development of a mature IBC is unknown.

During the formation of IBCs some *E. coli* differentiate to form filamentous bacteria. These are long filaments or snake-like bacteria that have been shown to form when cell division is blocked but growth continues [235]. Before *E. coli* exit uroepithelial cells, some bacteria regain their bacillary shape to become highly motile and exit the epithelial cell through disruptions in the cell membrane [233]. Filamentous bacteria have an advantage over their bacillary shaped counter parts, due to their elongated shaped which enhances their ability to avoid phagocytosis [236]. Filamentous bacteria have been identified in 41% of urine samples from women with a UTI, and of these 21% were observed to have exfoliated IBCs [237]. Whilst the transcriptional changes associated with filamentation are poorly understood, there is a strong suggestion that filamentous growth is a concerted response to host pressures [233].

Organisation and Regulation of Virulence Genes

Phase Variation of Type 1 Fimbriae and P pili

E. coli are able to control the expression of virulence genes depending on the environmental conditions and needs of the bacterium to create many different phenotypes [238]. Expression of type 1 fimbriae plays an important role early in the development of UTI (96). Within the first 24 hours of initiating infection in the bladder, the urinary bladder selects for the expression of type 1 fimbriae [239]. During cystitis, type 1 fimbriae are continually expressed in the bladder [85], however as *E. coli* move towards the kidney to cause pyelonephritis, expression is reduced via an invertible element that controls type 1 fimbriae switching to the 'off' position [239]. Among the regulatory genes, *fim*B is primarily the regulator that switches on the expression of type 1 fimbriae, and *fim*E acts to turn off the expression [240, 241]. P-fimbriae regulatory protein, PapB, reduces the expression of type 1 fimbriae by inhibiting the activity of FimB and increasing FimE activity, working together to switch the invertible element to the 'off' position [240, 241]. Once in the kidney, P-fimbriae is needed to attach to digalactoside receptors expressed on the kidney epithelium [242, 243]. The expression of genes responsible for the assembly and structure of type 1 fimbriae are co-regulated with P-fimbriae, with a bacterium expressing only one at a time [240, 241]. This may be a mechanism to help UPEC to conserve energy and resources [80]. Variable expression of these adhesins allows *E. coli* to successively colonize the bladder and kidney tissues [239, 244].

Mobile Genetic Elements

E. coli can acquire virulence properties that enhance their ability to cause UTI, and these specific genetic elements are often encoded in DNA segments called pathogenicity islands (PAIs) or in plasmids. Many virulence genes of UPEC are located on distinct insertions, such as plasmids or PAIs, and are less often located on the core genome [245]. Auxiliary genes involved in the assembly of pili or the excretion of toxins are often located on PAIs. These regions encode for clusters of virulence genes which contribute to the pathogenicity of UPEC. These regions are often unstable [245], with *E. coli* shown to lose their PAIs during growth in urine [246]. The acquisition of PAIs is a reversible process, whereby PAIs and the virulence factor that they encode can be lost again.

The evolution of new bacterial pathotypes is likely to begin with the integration of DNA into the bacterial genome. Bacterial plasmids are self-replicating extrachromosomal replicons that promote the distribution of various traits throughout bacterial populations [247]. *E. coli* can possess a range of plasmids encoding traits that can spread virulence, drug resistance, heavy metal resistance, metabolism of rare substances, and environmental adaptability and persistence amongst the population [248, 249]. Plasmids can harbor mobile genetic elements known as transposons and integrons, which can allow horizontal gene transfer between bacteria [249]. Plasmids are classified according to their incompatibility (Inc) with other plasmids, a phenomenon determined by their origin of replication (rep) [248, 249]. There are 26 known Inc or Rep groups as outlined in Table 2. Typing of these Inc groups allows a greater understanding of the dissemination and evolution of plasmids [250]. Some plasmids are unable to co-exist, either inhibiting transfer into the cell, or the loss of a plasmid overtime due to the unstable nature [249]. ExPEC are associated with plasmids encoding virulence and antimicrobial resistance [249]. Plasmid carrying virulence factors among UPEC primarily belonging to incompatibility family IncF [248, 249](Table 2). Two plasmids commonly associated with UPEC are the ColV and Vir plasmids. Whilst colicin V, which gives the ColV plasmids its name, is not associated with virulence, other factors conferred by this plasmid are associated with pathogenesis of UPEC [249]. This plasmid carries genes involved in iron acquisition and adherence, and has been associated with UTI and septicemia [249]. The Vir plasmid encodes a group of virulence factors, including cytotoxic necrotizing factor, that have the ability produce toxins and cause tissue damage [249].

There is generally a negative association between virulence genes and antibiotic resistance [251]. The FIB/FIIA plasmids often encode cytotoxic necrosing factor are frequently associated with *E. coli* causing UTI and septicemia [249, 252]. Of concern is the ability of repFIB/FIIA plasmids to acquire both virulence factors and multidrug resistant-encoding islands, which means they have the potential to provide selection for virulent strains through antibiotic therapy [249]. Bacterial plasmids have a high likelihood for transfer of antimicrobial resistance and the horizontal transfer of PAI sequences [253].

Table 2. Plasmid incompatibility (Inc) groups and their characteristics

Incompatibility Group	Characteristics
Com9, IncHI1, IncHI2, IncHI3, IncHII, IncI1, IncI2, IncK, IncL/M, IncR, IncU, IncV, IncX1, IncX2	Plasmids capable of carrying transfer and MDR function
IncA/C, IncN, IncP-α, IncP-β, IncP-γ, IncP-δ, IncP6 (IncG), IncP7, IncP9, IncQ	Broad-host-range plasmids capable of carrying transfer and MDR functions
IncB/O, IncFIB, IncFIC, IncFIIA, IncFIV, IncFV, IncFVI, IncFVII	Plasmids capable of carrying transfer, MDR, and virulence functions
IncD	Phage associated plasmids
IncJ	Conjugative, self-transmitting, integrating elements
IncQ1, IncQ2	Broad-host-range plasmids capable of carrying MDR functions
IncT	Large plasmids carrying transfer and DNA metabolism functions
IncY	Phage-like plasmids

Adapted from [249]. MDR: Multi drug resistance.

Evolution of Uropathogenic Virulence Factors

E. coli causing UTI differ from commensal strains by the presence of virulence genes, many of which are encoded by distinct insertions into the bacterial chromosome or on plasmids [254]. The diversity of virulence factors and the high level of genetic overlap between pathogenic and non-pathogenic *E. coli* makes it difficult to attribute a UPEC pathotype. Furthermore, UPEC have evolved multiple and redundant mechanisms to colonize the urinary tract [255], leaving no single feature to accurately define an isolate as UPEC. Some studies have suggested that virulence genes have evolved to help *E. coli* persist in the GI tract as resident flora, and the ability to cause UTI may be a coincidental consequence [6]. It is widely accepted that the GI tract is a major reservoir of UPEC, however whether the ability to cause infection is attributable to the prevalence of UPEC clones within the host (the prevalence hypothesis) or to the acquisition of virulence genes (the special-pathogenicity hypothesis) is widely debated. The prevalence theory suggests that the dominance of the causative UPEC strain within the GI tract is associated with an increased likelihood of migration to the urinary tract to cause UTI [256]. On the other hand, the special pathogenicity theory attributes the ability for UPEC to cause UTI to the selective advantage of the acquisition of virulence genes that have evolved to help UPEC colonize extraintestinal sites [257]. Although UPEC are predominant in the GI tract of healthy individuals [91], these strains must migrate to the urinary tract to cause UTI, meaning colonization of the GI tract is not sufficient to cause infection. In view of the prevalence of UPEC among healthy individuals, it has been suggested that virulence factors of UPEC have evolved to enhance intestinal colonization and/or transmission between hosts. In fact, both the dominance of UPEC in the GI tract and also the presence of uropathogenic virulence genes, have been shown to contribute to UTI [5].

UPEC Reservoirs

E. coli causing UTI are often characterized by the presence of multiple virulence factors which often make them genetically distinct from commensal strains of the GI tract [21]. Little is known about the origin of uropathogens. Molecular typing has enhanced our understanding of the modes of transmission and sources for infection. The fact that many UTIs in the community are caused by distinct strains suggests a reservoir in close proximity to the host, such as the vaginal area or GI tract [258]. It is well established that initial episodes of UTI are often caused by UPEC migrating from the GI tract and colonizing the vaginal area [259]. Following an initial episode, *E. coli* are able to persist within the bladder tissue, making the bladder a potential reservoir for UPEC [79]. From the bladder, UPEC are voided where they enter the environment to be passed to community sewage treatment plants, or re-introduced to the GI tract via a urine-oral route. Community-acquired UTIs are generally considered unrelated events and outbreaks caused by extraintestinal *E. coli* are not common, however there is mounting evidence for community-wide epidemics with examples found in California [260], London [261] and Copenhagen [262]. Analysis of these outbreaks has found no evidence of person-to-person transmission however, the limited available epidemiological data prevent definitive conclusions on potential food- or water- borne source [260-262]. Within households, *E. coli* are believed to be transmitted from person-to-person and between humans and pets [263-265].

Since the discovery of wide spread *E. coli* O25b-ST131 in 2008 [266, 267], this clonal group has rapidly become pandemic across multiple continents and has been implicated in various types of *E. coli* infections including UTI [268, 269]. Through the use of a public online multilocus sequence typing (MLST) database, the emergence of this clone can be dated back to 1992 with only sporadic incidence until the discovery of this clone in multiple countries in 2008 [266, 267]. ST131 is characterized by a high frequency of virulence genes and is frequently resistant to cephalosporin, fluroquinolones and trimethoprim, limiting antimicrobial therapeutic options for treatment of UTI [268]. This discovery of CTX-M-15 on the chromosome rather than plasmids is of concern, and may be a contributing factor for its global dissemination [267]. ST131 has been found in both human hosts and companion animals, which may have led to its wide dissemination [270, 271]. European studies have found ST131 to be predominant amongst uropathogenic isolates with up to 59% reported [268]. The prevalence of ST131 in the GI tract of healthy individuals, has received little attention [272]. In addition to ST131, other major sequence types (ST) causing UTI include ST-14, ST-69, ST-73, and ST-95. The dissemination of uropathogenic clones amongst the community and environment, including ST131, is poorly understood. These epidemics highlight the importance of understanding the mechanisms of UPEC transmission. Potential reservoirs of UPEC are discussed in more detail.

GI Tract Reservoirs

Little is known about the origin of uropathogens and their potential persistence in the GI tract of women prior to UTI. It has been found that up to 67% of recurrent UTIs are caused by the same *E. coli* strain, suggesting a reservoir for these strains enabling them to cause recurrent infections [5, 8, 273]. In recurrent episodes, the infecting strains has been found to be present in the faecal flora of 78% of women [8]. In acute cystitis episodes, 71% of patients have been shown to carry the UTI-causing strain as the dominant faecal clone [273]. It is unclear whether UPEC that migrate to cause UTI are selected because of their dominance in the GI tract, or because of the selective advantage provided by presence of virulence factors [5, 273]. The high number of uropathogenic virulence genes among human gastrointestinal isolates might reflex the adaptive nature needed for microflora to survive the changing nutritional environment of the human intestine. In a recent study, the GI tract of healthy humans has been identified as an important reservoir for carriage of UPEC, although this seems to be related to the age and gender of the host [91]. Furthermore, the presence of uropathogenic virulence genes being more frequently associated with *E. coli* isolated from the GI tract of humans rather than other mammals supports the hypothesis of the human intestine as a major reservoir of UPEC [18, 274].

Vaginal Reservoirs

Introital colonization provides a source for UPEC entry into the bladder. In women who experience frequent recurrent infections, colonization of the vaginal tract provides a constant reservoir of UPEC. In 68% of episodes of recurrent UTI, it has been found that the responsible pathogen established colonization of the vaginal introitus prior to causing infection [275, 276]. Vaginal epithelial cells cultured from women with recurrent UTI have been shown to support higher bacterial adherence, suggesting a host role in susceptibility to UTI [31]. Despite the role of the vaginal area in providing a reservoir for UPEC in the migration to the urinary tract, the presence of these uropathogens in these reservoirs is not associated with an increased risk of recurrent infection [38, 277], highlighting the role of the host in susceptibility to infection.

Bladder Reservoirs

Many recurrent UTIs are caused by the same strain responsible for the initial infection [44, 258]. Evidence over the past decade has shown that UPEC are able to invade bladder tissues and latently persist for months within vesicles as quiescent intracellular reservoirs (QIRs) [278]. In a mouse model of UTI, UPEC have been shown to invade the bladder epithelium and survive for months following an initial UTI [83]. In response to infection the apical epithelial cells are shed and exfoliated into the urine, exposing deeper tissue layers, and some UPEC are able to gain access and infect the underlying basal epithelium. Within these immature bladder cells, UPEC persist in vacuoles enmeshed in a network of actin fibers to establish a quiescent intracellular reservoir (QIR). UPEC can remain dormant in QIRs where they can persist undetected from the host immune system for months [278]. UPEC in QIRs are also protected from antibiotic treatments, many of which are effective against actively growing bacteria. The bladder has slow turnover rate [29], which may be a contributing factor for the ability of UPEC to remains as intracellular reservoirs longer after clinical symptoms have subsided [76, 80]. Terminal differentiation of immature bladder epithelial cells as they migrate to the luminal surface of the bladder, leads to the reorganization of F-actin, allowing the release of UPEC from their vacuoles, leading to bacterial replication and formation of new IBCs and relapse infection [77]. The establishment of QIRs is considered a major reservoir of recurrent infections among women.

Environmental Reservoirs

E. coli exists as part of the normal microflora of the human intestines, however once expelled it becomes a potential biological hazard in environmental waters. A majority of these *E. coli* do not survive in the environment due to changes in temperature, sedimentation and nutrient availability and the bactericidal effects of UV sunlight [279, 280]. Of concern is the presence of *E. coli* with uropathogenic virulence genes in final effluent of sewage treatment plants, and their release into surrounding water ways [281]. These results indicate that uropathogen dissemination is common amongst humans and the environment. The role of uropathogenic virulence factors for enhancing environmental survival remains to be determined.

Given our understanding of *E. coli* in the environment, the potential exists for the spread UPEC through the faecal-oral route via contamination of food and water. In fact, foodborne transmission has been implicated in the dissemination of *E. coli* causing community-acquired UTI [282]. Birds in particular have been shown to harbor large amounts of *E. coli* carrying common uropathogenic virulence genes [274, 283]. Animal to human transmission of bacteria can occur in people who are in frequent contact with animals such as pig farmers [284]. A potential link between animal, surface waters and food sources of UPEC is a major public health concern and highlights the importance and needs further investigation.

Conclusion

Despite much research into the pathogenesis of UPEC, UTI remains one of the most common infectious diseases among hospitalized patients worldwide. Horizontal gene transfer will continuously offer up new bacterial pathotypes. The larger genome of UPEC compared to commensal strain suggests that there remains many uncharacterised uropathogenic virulence factors. This chapter has discussed virulence factors that promote *E. coli* persistence in the GI and urinary tracts. Information on virulence gene profiles of *E. coli* causing UTI among susceptible patient groups, such as children and postmenopausal women, is limited. Further research into quiescent intracellular reservoir as well as persistence of UPEC in the GI tract of patients with UTI and their reappearance in the GI tract after antibiotic therapy may reveal why some women experience recurrent UTIs. UPEC employ complex, multifaceted strategies to colonize and survive the harsh physiological environment of the bladder. Virulence genes enhance the ability of UPEC to adhere, colonize and survive in the urinary tract, increasing the pathogenicity of these bacteria. These virulence factors may be potential targets for future drug therapies to immobilize essential bacterial virulence mechanism for future treatment of UTI. *E. coli* carrying uropathogenic properties are normally present and may dominate the faecal flora, thus factors that promote their intestinal colonization is also of importance in the preventing development of UTI by these bacteria.

References

[1] Law D (1994) Adhesion and its role in the virulence of enteropathogenic *Escherichia coli. Clin Micro Rev* 7 (2):152-173.

[2] Campbell NA, Reece JB (2002) Biology. Pearson Education Inc, San Francisco.

[3] Kaper JB, Nataro JP, Mobley HLT (2004) Pathogenic *Escherichia coli. Nat Rev Microbiol* 2:123-140.

[4] Salyers AA, Whitt DD (2002) Bacterial pathogenesis: a molecular approach. ASM Press, Washington DC.

[5] Moreno E, Andreu A, Pigrau C, Kuskowski MA, Johnson JR, Prats G (2008) Relationship between *Escherichia coli* strains causing acute cystitis in women and the fecal *E. coli* population of the host. *J Clin Microbiol* 46 (8):2529-2534.

[6] Tullus K, Kühn I, Ørskov I, Ørskov F, Möllby R (1992) The importance of P and type 1 fimbriae for the persistence of *Escherichia coli* in the human gut. *Epidemiol Infect* 108 (3):415-421.

[7] Schlager TA, Hendley JO, Bell AL, Whittam TS (2002) Clonal diversity of *Escherichia coli* colonizing stools and urinary tracts of young girls. *Infect Immun* 70 (3):1225-1229.

[8] Czaja CA, Stamm WE, Stapleton AE, Roberts PL, Hawn TR, Scholes D, Samadpour M, Hultgren SJ, Hooton TM (2009) Prospective cohort study of microbial and inflammatory events immediately preceding *Escherichia coli* recurrent urinary tract infection in women. *J Infect Dis* 200 (4):528-536.

[9] Obata-Yasuoka M, Ba-Thein W, Tsukamoto T, Yoshikawa H, Hayashi H (2002) Vaginal *Escherichia coli* share common virulence factor profiles, serotypes and phylogeny with other extraintestinal *E. coli*. *Microbiology* 148:2745-2752.

[10] Albanese CT, Smith SD, Watkins S, Kurkchubasche A, Simmons RL, Rowe MI (1994) Effect of secretory IgA on transepithelial passage of bacteria across the intact ileum in vitro. *J Am Coll Surg* 179 (6):679-688.

[11] Guarner F, Malagelada J (2003) Gut flora in health and disease. *The Lancet* 360:512-519.

[12] Albanese CT, Cardona M, Smith SD, Watkins S, Kurkchubasche AG, Ulman I, Simmons RL, Rowe MI (1994) Role of intestinal mucus in transepithelial passage of bacteria across the intact ileum in vitro. *Surgery* 116 (1):76-82.

[13] Bollinger RR, Everett ML, Palestrant D, Love SD, Lin SS, Parker W (2003) Human secretory immunoglobulin A may contribute to biofilm formation in the gut. *Immunology* 109:580-587.

[14] Penders J, Thijs C, Vink C, Stelma FF, Snijders B, Kummeling I, vandenBrandt PA, Stobberingh EE (2006) Factors influencing the composition of the intestinal microbiotia in early infancy. *Pediatrics* 118 (2):511-521.

[15] Gronlund MM, Lehtonen OP, Eerola E, Kero P (1999) Faecal microflora in healthy infants born by different methods of delivery: permanent changes in intestinal flora after caesarean delivery. *J Pediatr Gatroenterol Nutr* 29:19-25.

[16] Harmsen HJ, Wildeboer-Veloo AC, Raangs GC, Wagendorp AA, Klijn JG, Bindels JG, Welling GW (2000) Analysis of intestinal flora development in breast-fed and formula-fed by using molecular identification detection methods. *J Pediatr Gatroenterol Nutr* 30:61-67.

[17] Sakata H, Yoshioka H, Fujita K (1984) Development of the intestinal flora in very low birth weight infants compared to normal full-term newborns. *Europ J Pediatr* 144:186-190.

[18] Tenaillon O, Skurnik D, Picard B, Denamur E (2010) The population genetics of commensal *Escherichia coli*. *Nat Rev Microbiol* 8:207-217.

[19] Nowrouzian FL, Wold AE, Adlerberth I (2005) *Escherichia coli* strains belonging to phylogenetic group B2 have superior capacity to persist in the intestinal microflora of infants. *J Infect Dis* 191 (7):1078-1083.
[20] Nowrouzian F, Adlerberth I, Wold AE (2001) P fimbriae, capsule and aerobactin characterize colonic resident *Escherichia coli. Epidemiol Infect* 126:11-18.
[21] Johnson JR (1991) Virulence factors in *Escherichia coli* urinary tract infection. *Clin Micro Rev* 4 (1):80-128.
[22] Pfau A, Sacks T (1981) The bacterial flora of the vaginal vestibule, urethra and vagina in premenopausal women with recurrent urinary tract infections. *J Urol* 126:630-634.
[23] Krohn MA, Thwin SS, Rabe LK, Brown Z, Hillier SL (1997) Vaginal colonization by *Escherichia coli* as a risk factor for very low birth weight delivery and other perinatal complications. *J Infect Dis* 175:606-610.
[24] Sarff LD, McCracken GH, Schiffer MS, Glode MP, Robbins JB, Orskov I, Orskov F (1975) Epidemiology of *Escherichia coli* K1 in healthy and diseased newborns. *Lancet* 1 (7916):1099-1104.
[25] Stamey TA, Sexton CC (1975) The role of vaginal colonization with Enterobacteriaceae in recurrent urinary tract infections. *J Urol* 113:214-217.
[26] Stamey TA, Timothy M, Millar M, Mihara G (1971) Recurrent urinary infections in adult women. The role of introital enterobacteria. *Calif Med* 115 (1-19).
[27] Boskey ER, Telsch KM, Whaley KJ, Moench TR, Cone RA (1999) Acid production by vaginal flora in vitro is consistent with the rate and extent of vaginal acidification. *Infect Immun* 67 (10):5170-5175.
[28] Schaefer AJ, Stamey TA (1977) Studies of introital colonization in women with recurrent urinary infections. IX. The role of antimicrobial therapy. *J Urol* 118:221-224.
[29] Apodaca G (2004) The uroepithelium: not just a passive barrier. *Traffic* 5 (3):117-128.
[30] Klumpp DJ, Forrestal SG, Karr JE, Mudge CS, Anderson BE, Schaeffer AJ (2002) Epithelial differentiation promotes the adherence of type 1-piliated *Escherichia coli* to human vaginal cells. *J Infect Dis* 186:1631-1638.
[31] Schaeffer AJ, Jones JM, Dunn JK (1981) Association of vitro *Escherichia coli* adherence to vaginal and buccal epithelial cells with

susceptibility of women to recurrent urinary-tract infections. *N Engl J Med* 304:1062-1066.

[32] Marrie T, Swantee C, Hartlen M (1980) Aerobic and anaerobic urethral flora of healthy females in various physiological age groups and of females with urinary tract infections. *J Clin Microbiol* 11:654-659.

[33] Murray PR, Rosenblatt JE (1976) Bacterial interference by oropharyngeal and clinical isolates of anaerobic bacteria. *J Infect Dis* 134:281-285.

[34] Foxman B, Chi JW (1990) Health behavior and urinary tract infection in college-aged women. *J Clin Epidemiol* 43:329-337.

[35] Strom BL, Collins M, West SL, Kreisberg J, Weller S (1987) Sexual activity, contraceptive use, and other risk factors for symptomatic and asymptomatic bacteriuria. *Ann Intern Med* 107:816-823.

[36] Fihn SD, Johnson C, Pinkstaff C, Stamm WE (1986) Diaphragm use and urinary tract infections: analysis of urodynamic and microbiological factors. *J Urol* 136:853-856.

[37] Hooton TM, Fennel CL, Clark AM, Stamm WE (1991) Nonoxynol-9: differential antiacterial activity and enhancement of bacterial activity and enhancement of bacterial adherence to vaginal epithelial cells. *J Infect Dis* 164:1216-1219.

[38] Stapleton A, Hooton TM, Fennell C, Roberts PL, Stamm WE (1995) Effect of secretor status on vaginal and rectal colonization with fimbriated *Escherichia coli* in women with and without recurrent urinary tract infection. *J Infect Dis* 171 (717-729).

[39] Stapleton A, Nudelman E, Clausen H, Hakomori S, Stamm WE (1992) Binding of uropathogenic *Escherichia coli* R45 to glycolipids extracted from vaginal epithelial cells is dependent on histo-blood group secretor status. *J Clin Invest* 90:965-972.

[40] Stapleton AE, Stroud MR, Hakomori SI, Stamm WE (1998) The globoseries glycosphingolipid sialosyl galactosyl globoside is found in urinary tract tissues and is a preferred binding receptor In vitro for uropathogenic *Escherichia coli* expressing *pap*-encoded adhesins. *Infect Immun* 66 (8):3856-3861.

[41] Ishitoya S, Yamamoto K, Mitsumori K, Ogawa O, Terai A (2002) Non-secretor status is associated with female acute uncomplicated pyelonephritis. *BJU Int* 89:851-854.

[42] Raz R (2011) Urinary tract infection in postmenopausal women. Korean J Urol 52:801-808.

[43] Gameiro CM, Romão F, Castelo-Branco C (2010) Menopause and aging: changes in the immune system—a review. *Maturitas* 67 (4):316-320.

[44] Ikäheimo R, Siitonen A, Heiskanen T, Kärkkäinen U, Kuosmanen P, Leipponen P, Mäkelä PH (1996) Recurrence of urinary tract infection in a primary care setting: analysis of a 1-year follow-up of 179 women. *Clin Infect Dis* 22 (1):91-99.

[45] Wira CR, Fahey JV, Ghosh M, Patel MV, Hickey DK, Ochiel DO (2010) Sex hormone regulation of innate immunity in the female reproductive tract: The role of epithelial cells in balancing reproductive potential with protection against sexually transmitted pathogens. *Am J Reprod Immunol* 63:544-565.

[46] Raz R, Stamm WE (1993) A controlled trial of intravaginal estriol in postmenopausal women with recurrent urinary tract infections. *New Engl J Med* 329 (11):753-756.

[47] Lüthje P, Brauner H, Ramos NL, Ovregaard A, Gläser R, Hirscherberg AL, Aspenström P, Brauner A (2013) Estrogen supports urothelial defense mechanisms. *Sci Transl Med* 5 (190):190ra180.

[48] Chromek M, Brauner A (2008) Antimicrobial mechanisms of the urinary tract. *J Med Microbiol* 86:37-47.

[49] Carbonetti NH, Bonnchai S, Parry SH, Väisänen-Rhen V, Korhonen TK, Williams PH (1986) Aerobactin-mediated iron uptake by *Escherichia coli* isolates from human extraintestinal infections. *Infect Immun* 51 (3):966-968.

[50] De Brito BG, da Silvia Leite D, Linhares REC, Vidotto MC (1999) Virulence-associated factors of uropathogenic *Escherichia coli* strains isolated from pigs. *Vet Microbiol* 65:123-132.

[51] Fletcher J (1971) The effect of iron and transferrin on the killing of *Escherichia coli* in fresh serum. *Immunology* 20:493-500.

[52] Opal SM, Cross AS, Gemski P, Lyhte LW (1990) Aerobactin and α-hemolysin as virulence determinants in *Escherichia coli* isolated from human blood, urine, and stool. *J Infect Dis* 161 (4):794-796.

[53] Russo TA, Carlino UB, Mong A, Jodush ST (1999) Identification of genes in an extraintestinal isolate of *Escherichia coli* with increased expression after exposure to human urine. *Infect Immun* 67 (10):5306-5314.

[54] Abrink M, Larsson E, Gobl A, Hellman L (2000) Expression of lactoferrin in the kidney: Implications for innate immunity and iron metabolism. *Kidney Int* 57 (5):2004-2010.

[55] Drago-Serrano ME, de la Garza-Amaya M, Luna JS, Campos-Rodríguez R (2012) Lactoferrin-lipopolysaccharide (LPS) binding as key to antibacterial and antiendotoxic effects. *Int Immunopharmacol* 12 (1):1-9.

[56] Johnson JR, Moseley SL, Roberts PL, Stamm WE (1988) Aerobactin and other virulence factor genes among strains of *Escherichia coli* causing urosepsis: association with patient characteristics. *Infect Immun* 56 (2):405-412.

[57] Kim KS, Itabashi H, Gemski P, Sadoff J, Warren RL, Cross AS (1992) The K1 capsule is the critical determinant in the development of *Escherichia coli* meningitis in the rat. *J Clin Invest* 90 (3):897-905.

[58] Dhakal BK, Kulesus RR, Mulvey MA (2008) Mechanisms and consequences of bladder cell invasion by uropathogenic *Escherichia coli*. *Eur J Clin Invest* 38:2-11.

[59] Eto DS, Jones TA, Sundsbak JL, Mulvey MA (2007) Integrin-mediated host cell invasion by type 1-piliated uropathogenic *Escherichia coli*. *PLoS Pathogen* 3 (7):949-961.

[60] Jones CH, Pinkner JS, Roth R, Heuser J, Nicholes AV, Abraham SN, Hultgren SJ (1995) FimH adhesin of type 1 pili is assembled into a fibrillar tip structure in the *Enterobacteriaceae*. *P Natl Acad Sci* 92:2081-2085.

[61] Arthur M, Johnson CE, Rubin RH, Arbeit RD, Campanelli C, Kim C, Steinbach S, Agarwal M, Wilkinson R, Goldstein R (1989) Molecular epidemiology of adhesin and hemolysin virulence factors among uropathogenic *Escherichia coli*. *Infect Immun* 57 (2):303-313.

[62] Holden NJ, Gally DL (2004) Switches, cross-talk and memory in *Escherichia coli* adherence. *J Med Microbiol* 53:585-593.

[63] Giampapa CS, Abraham SN, Chiang TM, Beachey EH (1988) Isolation and characterization of a receptor for type 1 fimbriae of *Escherichia coli* from guinea pig erythrocytes. *J Biol Chem* 263 (11):5362-5367.

[64] Wold AE, Mestecky J, Tomana M, Kobata A, Ohbayashi H, Endo T, SvanborgEdén C (1990) Secretory immunoglobulin A carries oligosaccharide receptors for *Escherichia coli* type 1 fimbrial lectin. *Infect Immun* 58 (9):3073-3077.

[65] Sokurenko EV, Courtney HS, Ohman DE, Klemm P, Hasty DL (1994) FimH family of type 1 fimbrial adhesins: functional heterogeneity due to minor sequence variations among *fimH* genes. *J Bacteriol* 176 (3):748-755.

[66] Zhou G, Mo W-J, Sebbel P, Min G, Neubert TA, Glockshuber R, Wu X-R, Sun T-T, Kong X-P (2001) Uroplakin Ia is the urothelial receptor for

uropathogenic *Escherichia coli*: evidence from in vitro FimH binding. *J Cell Sci* 114 (22):4095-4103.

[67] Wold AE, Thorssén M, Hull S, SvanborgEdén C (1988) Attachment of *Escherichia coli* via mannose- or Galα1→ 4Galβ- containing receptors to human colonic epithelial cells. *Infect Immun* 56 (10):2531-2537.

[68] Falkowski W, Edwards M, Schaeffer AJ (1986) Inhibitory effect of substituted aromatic hydrocarbons on adherence of *Escherichia coli* to human epithelial cells. *Infect Immun* 52:863-866.

[69] Chowdhury P, Sacks SH, Sheerin NS (2004) Functions of the renal tract epithelium in coordinating the innate immune response to infection. *Kidney Int* 66:1334-1340.

[70] Virkola R, Westerlund B, Holthöfer H, Parkkinen J, Kekomäki M, Korhonen TK (1988) Binding characteristics of *Escherichia coli* adhesins in human urinary bladder. *Infect Immun* 56 (10):2615-2622.

[71] Saemann MD, Weichhart T, Horl WH, Zlabinger GJ (2005) Tamm-Horsfall protein: a multilayered defence molecule against urinary tract infection. *Eur J Clin Invest* 35:227-235.

[72] Sivick KE, Mobley HLT (2010) Waging war against uropathogenic *Escherichia coli*: winning back the urinary tract. *Infect Immun* 78 (2):568-585.

[73] Mak RH, Kuo H-J (2006) Pathogenesis of urinary tract infection: an update. *Curr Opin Pediatr* 18:148-152.

[74] Thomas WE, Nilsson LM, Forero M, Sokurenko EV, Vogel V (2004) Shear-dependent "stick-and-roll" adhesion of type 1 fimbriated *Escherichia coli*. *Mol Microbiol* 53:1545-1557.

[75] Abraham SN, Shin JS, Malaviya R (2001) Type 1 fimbriated *Escherichia coli* - Mast cell interactions in cystitis. *J Infect Dis* 183 (Suppl 1):S51- S55.

[76] Mulvey MA, Schilling JD, Hultgren SJ (2001) Establishment of a persistent *Escherichia coli* reservoir during acute phase of a bladder infection. *Infect Immun* 69:4572-4579.

[77] Eto DS, Sundsbak JL, Mulvey MA (2006) Actin-gated intracellular growth and resurgence of uropathogenic *Escherichia coli*. *Cell Microbiol* 8 (4):704-717.

[78] Palmer LM, Reilly TJ, Utsalo SJ, Donnenberg MS (2007) Internalization of *E. coli* by human renal epithelial cells is associated with tyrosine phosphorylation of specific host proteins. *Infect Immun* 65:2570-2575.

[79] Anderson GG, Palermo JJ, Schilling JD, Roth R, Heuser J, Hultgren SJ (2003) Intracellular bacterial biofilm-like pods in urinary tract infections. *Science* 301:105-107.

[80] Mulvey MA (2002) Adhesion and entry of uropathogenic *Escherichia coli*. *Cellular Microbiol* 4 (5):257-271.

[81] Mysorekar IU, Mulvey MA, Hultgren SJ, Gordon JI (2002) Molecular regulation of urothelial renewal and host defenses during infection with uropathogenic *Escherichia coli*. *J Biol Chem* 277 (9):7412-7419.

[82] Southgate J, Kennedy W, Hutton KAR, Trejdosiewicz LK (1995) Expression and *in vitro* regulation of integrins by normal human urothelial cells. *Cell Adhes Commun* 3 (3):231-242.

[83] Mulvey MA, Lopez-Boado YS, Wilson CL, Roth R, Parks WC, Heuser J, Hultgren SJ (1998) Induction and evasion of host defenses by type 1-piliated uropathogenic *Escherichia coli*. *Science* 282 (5393):1494-1497.

[84] Berry RE, Klumpp DJ, Schaeffer AJ (2009) Urothelial cultures support intracellular bacterial community formation by uropathogenic *Escherichia coli*. *Infect Immun* 77 (7):2762-2772.

[85] Connell H, Agace W, Klemm P, Schembri M, Mårild S, Svanborg C (1996) Type 1 fimbrial expression enhances *Escherichia coli* virulence for the urinary tract. *Proc Natl Acad Sci USA* 93:9827-9832.

[86] Hung CS, Bouckaert J, Hung D, Pinkner J, Widberg C, DeFusco A (2002) Structural basis of tropism of *Escherichia coli* to the bladder during urinary tract infection. *Mol Microbiol* 44:903-915.

[87] Sokurenko EV, Courtney HS, Maslow J, Siitonen A, Hasty DI (1995) Quantitative differences in adhesiveness of type 1 fimbriated *Escherichia coli* due to structural differences in *fimH* genes. *J Bacteriol* 177 (13):3680-3686.

[88] Pouttu R, Puustinen T, Virkola R, Hacker J, Klemm P, Korhonen TK (1999) Amino acid residue Ala-62 in the FimH fimbrial adhesin is critical for the adhesiveness of meningitis-associated *Escherichia coli* to collagens. *Mol Microbiol* 31:1747-1757.

[89] Sokurenko EV, Chesnokova V, Doyle RJ, Hasty DL (1997) Diversity of the *Escherichia coli* type 1 fimbrial lectin. Differential binding to mannosides and uroepithelial cells. *J Biol Chem* 272:17880-17886.

[90] Duguid JP, Gillies RR (1957) Fimbriae and adhesive properties in dysenteric bacilli. *J Pathol Bacteriol* 74:397-401.

[91] Vollmerhausen TL, Ramos NL, Gündoğdu A, Robinson W, Brauner A, Katouli M (2011) Population structure and uropathogenic virulence-

associated genes of fecal *Escherichia coli* of healthy young and elderly adults. *J Med Microbiol* 60:574-581.

[92] Wold AE, Caugant DA, Lidin-Janson G, deMan P, Svanborg C (1992) Resident colonic *Escherichia coli* strains frequently display uropathogenic characteristics. *J Infect Dis* 165:46-52.

[93] Snyder J, Haugen B, Lockatell CV, Maroncle N, Hagan EC, Johnson DE, Welch RA, Mobley HLT (2005) Coordinate expression of fimbriae in uropathogenic *Escherichia coli. Infect Immun* 73 (11):7588-7596.

[94] Silverblatt FJ, Dreyer JS, Schauer S (1979) Effect of pili on susceptibility of *Escherichia coli* to phagocyctosis. *Infect Immun* 24 (1):218-223.

[95] Plos K, Connell H, Jodal U, Marklund B, Mårild S, Wettergren B, Svanborg C (1995) Intestinal carriage of P fimbriated *Escherichia coli* and the susceptibility to urinary tract infection in young children. *J Infect Dis* 171:625-631.

[96] Holden NJ, Totsika M, Mahler E, Roe AJ, Catherwood K, Lindner K, Dobrindt U, Gally DL (2006) Demonstration of regulatory cross-talk between P fimbriae and type 1 fimbriae in uropathogenic *Escherichia coli. Microbiology* 152:1143-1153.

[97] GuntherIV NW, Snyder JA, Lockatell V, Blomfield I, Johnson DE, Mobley HLT (2002) Assessment of virulence of uropathogenic *Escherichia coli* type 1 fimbrial mutants in which the invertible element is phase-lock on or off. *Infect Immun* 70 (7):3344-3354.

[98] Svanborg Edén C, Fasth A, Hagberg L, Hanson LÅ, Korhonen T, Leffler H (1982) Host interaction with *Escherichia coli* in the urinary tract. *Semin Infect Dis* 4:113-131.

[99] Kallenius G, Mollby R (1979) Adhesion of *Escherichia coli* to human periurethral cells correlated to mannose-resistant agglutination of human erythrocytes. *FEMS Microbiol Lett* 5:295-299.

[100] Bock K, Breimer ME, Hansson GC, Karlsson KA, Larson G, Leffler H, Samuelsson BE, Strömberg N, Edén CS (1985) Specificity of binding of a strain of uropathogenic *Escherichia coli* to Gal alpha 1----4Gal-containing glycosphingolipids. *J Biol Chem* 260 (14):8545-8551.

[101] Björnham O, Nilsson H, Andersson M, Schedin S (2009) Physical properties of the specific PapG-galabiose binding in *E. coli* P pili-mediated adhesion. *Eur Biophys J* 38:245-254.

[102] Johnson JR (1998) *papG* alleles among *Escherichia coli* strains causing urosepsis: associations with other bacterial characteristics and host compromise. *Infect Immun* 66 (9):4568-4571.

[103] Tseng C, Huang J, Wang M, Wu A, Ko W, Chen W, Wu J (2007) PapG II adhesin in the establishment and persistence of *Escherichia coli* infection in mouse kidneys. *Kidney Int* 71:764-770.

[104] Kuehn MJ, Heuser J, Normark S, Hultgren SJ (1992) P pili in uropathogneic *E. coli* are composite fibres with distinct fibrillar adhesive tips. *Nature* 356 (6366):252-255.

[105] Zhano L, Chen X, Zhu X, Yang W, Dong L, Xu X, Gao S, Lui X (2009) Prevalence of virulence factors and antimicrobial resistance of uropathogenic *Escherichia coli* in Jiangsu province (China). *Urology* 74 (3):702-707.

[106] Lane MC, Mobley M (2007) Role of P-fimbrial-mediated adherence in pyelonephritis and persistence of uropathogenic *Escherichia coli* (UPEC) in the mammalian kidney. *Kidney Int* 72:19-25.

[107] Johnson JR, Russo TA, Brown JJ, Stapleton A (1998) *papG* alleles of *Escherichia coli* strains causing first episode or recurrent acute cystitis in adult women. *J Infect Dis* 177:97-101.

[108] Ewers C, Antao EM, Diehl I, Philipp HC, Wieler LH (2009) Intestine and environment of the chicken as reservoirs for extraintestinal pathogenic *Escherichia coli* strains with zoonotic potential. *Appl Environ Microbiol* 75 (1):184-192.

[109] Hedlund M, Svensson M, Nilsson A, Duan RD, Svanborg C (1996) Role of the ceramide-signaling pathway in cytokine responses to P-fimbriated *Escherichia coli*. *J Exp Med* 183 (3):1037-1044.

[110] Fischer H, Ellström P, Ekström K, Gustafsson L, Gustafsson M, Svanborg C (2007) Ceramide as a TLR4 agonist; A putative signalling intermediate between sphingolipid receptors for microbial ligands and TLR4. *Cell Microbiol* 9 (5):1239-1251.

[111] Bergsten G, Wullt B, Svanborg C (2005) *Escherichia coli*, fimbriae, bacterial persistence and host response induction in the human urinary tract. *Int J Med Microbio*l 296:487-502.

[112] Tewari R, Ikeda T, Malaviya R, MacGregor JI, Little JR, Hultgren SJ, Abraham SN (1994) The PapG tip adhesin of P fimbriae protects *Escherichia coli* from neutrophil bactericidal activity. *Infect Immun* 62 (12):5296-5304.

[113] Rice JC, Peng T, Spence JA, Wang H-Q, Goldblum RM, Corthesy B, Nowicki BJ (2005) Pyelonephritic Escherichia coli expressing P fimbriae decrease immune response of the mouse kidney. *J Am Soc Nephrol* 16:3583-3591.

[114] Nowrouzian F, Wold AE, Adlerberth I (2001) P fimbriae and aerobactin as intestinal colonization factors for *Escherichia coli* in Pakistani infants. Epidemiol Infect 126:19-23.

[115] Svanborg Edén C, Eriksson B, Hanson LÅ (1977) Adhesion of *Escherichia coli* to human uroepithelial cells in vitro. *Infect Immun* 18:767-774.

[116] Parkkinen J, Finne J, Achtman M, Vaisanen V, Korhonen TK (1983) *Escherichia coli* strains binding neuraminyl alpha 2-3 galactosides. *Biochem Biophys Res Commun* 111 (2):456-461.

[117] Malagolini N, Cavallone D, Wu XR, Serafini-Cessi F (2000) Terminal glycosylation of bovine uroplakin III, one of the major integral-membrane glycoproteins of mammalian bladder. *Biochem Biophys Acta* 1475:231-237.

[118] Morschhauser J, Vetter V, Korhonen T, Uhlin BE, Hacker J (1993) Regulation and binding properties of S fimbriae cloned from *E. coli* strains causing urinary tract infection and meningitis. *Zentralbl Bakteriol* 278 (2-3):165-176.

[119] Marre R, Hacker J, Henkel W, Goebel W (1986) Contribution of cloned virulence factors from uropathogenic *Escherichia coli* strains to nephropathogenicity in an experimental rat pyelonephritis model. *Infect Immun* 54 (3):761-767.

[120] Hacker J, Kestler H, Hoschutzky H, Jann K, Lottspeich F, Korhonen TK (1993) Cloning and characterization of the S fimbrial adhesin II complex of an *Escherichia coli* O18: K1 meningitis isolate. *Infect Immun* 61:544-550.

[121] Johnson TJ, Wannemuehler Y, Johnson SJ, Stell AL, Doetkott C, Johnson JR, Kim KS, Spanjaard L, Nolan LK (2008) Comparison of extraintestinal pathogenic *Escherichia coli* strains from human and avian sources reveals a mixed subset representing potential zoonotic pathogens. *Appl Environ Microbiol* 74 (22):7043-7050.

[122] Riegman N, Kusters R, Van Veggel H, Bergmans H, Van Bergen en Henegouwen P, Hacker J, Van Die I (1990) F1C fimbriae of a uropathogenic *Escherichia coli* strain: genetic and functional organization of the foc gene cluster and identification of minor subunits. *J Bacteriol* 172 (2):1114-1120.

[123] Ott M, Hoschutzky H, Jann K, Van Die I, Hacker J (1988) Gene clusters for S fimbrial adhesin (*sfa*) and F1C fimbriae (*foc*) of *Escherichia coli*: comparative aspects structure function. *J Bacteriol* 170:3983-3990.

[124] Khan AS, Kniep B, Oelschlaeger TA, Van Die I, Korhonen T, Hacker J (2000) Receptor structure for F1C fimbriae of uropathogenic *Escherichia coli. Infect Immun* 68:3541-3547.

[125] Siitonen A, Martikainen R, Ikäheimo R, Palmgren J, Mäkelä PH (1993) Virulence-associated characteristics of *Escherichia coli* in urinary tract infection: a statistical analysis with special attention to type 1C fimbriation. *Microb Pathog* 15 (1):65-75.

[126] Lasaro MA, Salinger N, Zhang J, Wang Y, Zhong Z, Goulian M, Zhu J (2009) F1C fimbriae play an important role in biofilm formation and intestinal colonisation by the *Escherichia coli* commensal strain Nissle 1917. *Appl Environ Microbiol* 75 (1):246-251.

[127] Goluszko P, Selvarangan R, Nowicki BJ, Nowicki S, Hart A, Pawelczyk E, Nguyen K (2001) Rapid receptor-clustering assay to detect uropathogenic and diarrheal *Escherichia coli* isolates bearing adhesins of the DR family. *J Clin Microbiol* 39 (6):2317-2320.

[128] Foxman B, Zhang L, Tallman P, Palin K, Rode C, Bloch C, Gillespie B, Marrs CF (1995) Virulence characteristics of *Escherichia coli* causing first urinary tract infection predict risk of second infection. *J Infect Dis* 172 (6):1536-1541.

[129] Nowicki B, Selvarangan R, Nowicki S (2001) Family of *Escherichia coli* DR adhesins: decay-accelerating factor receptor recognition and invasiveness. *J Infect Dis* 183 (Suppl 1):S24-S27.

[130] Johnson JR, Owens K, Gajewski A, Kuskowski MA (2005) Bacterial characteristics in relation to clinical source of *Escherichia coli* isolates from women with acute cystitis or pyelonephritis and uninfected women. *J Clin Microbiol* 43 (12):6064-6072.

[131] Goluszko P, Niesel D, Nowicki B, Selvarangan R, Nowicki S, Hart A, Pawelczyke E, Das M, Urvil P, Hasan R (2001) DR operon-associated invasiveness of *Escherichia coli* from pregnant patients with pyelonephritis. *Infect Immun* 69 (7):4678-4680.

[132] Tieng V, Le Bouguénec D, du Merle L, Bertheau P, Desreumaux P, Janin A, Charron D, Toubert A (2002) Binding of *Escherichia coli* adhesin AfaE to CD55 triggers cell-surface expression of the MHC class I-related molecule MICA. *Proc Natl Acad Sci USA* 5 (99):2977-2982.

[133] Bilge SS, Clausen CR, Lau W, Moseley SL (1989) Molecular characterisation of a fimbrial adhesin, F1845, mediating diffuse adherence of diarrhea-associated *Escherichia coli* to HEp-2 cells. *J Bacteriol* 171:4281-4289.

[134] Ejrnaes K, Stegger M, Reisner A, Ferry S, Monsen T, Holm SE, Lundgren B, Frimodt-Møller N (2011) Characteristics of *Escherichia coli* causing persistence or relapse of urinary tract infections: phylogenetic groups, virulence factors and biofilm formation. *Virulence* 2 (6):1-10.

[135] Schembri MA, Klemm P (2001) Coordinate gene regulation by fimbriae-induced signal transduction. *EMBO J* 20 (12):3074-3081.

[136] Danese PN, Pratt LA, Dove SL, Kilter R (2000) The outer membrane protein, Antigen 43, mediates cell-to-cell interactions within *Escherichia coli* biofilms. *Mol Microbiol 3*7 (2):424-432.

[137] Ulett GC, Valle J, Beloin C, Sherlock O, Ghigo J-M, Schembri MA (2007) Functional analysis of antigen 43 in uropathogenic *Escherichia coli* reveals a role in long-term persistence in the urinary tract. *Infect Immun* 75 (7):3233-3244.

[138] Stoodley P, Sauer K, Davies DG, Costerton JW (2002) Biofilms as complex differentiated communities. Annu Rev Microbiol 56:187-209.

[139] Donlan RM (2002) Biofilms: microbial life on surfaces. *Emerg Infect Dis* 8 (9):881-890.

[140] Costerton JW, Stewart PS, Greenberg EP (1999) Bacterial biofilms: a common cause of persistent infections. *Science* 284:1318-1322.

[141] Yildiz FH, Schoolnik GK (1999) *Vibrio cholerae* O1 El Tor: Identification of a gene cluster required for the rugose colony type, exopolysaccharide production, chlorine resistance, and biofilm formation. *Proc Natl Acad Sci USA* 96 (7):4028-4033.

[142] Schembri MA, Kjærgaard K, Klemm P (2003) Global gene expression in *Escherichia coli* biofilms. *Mol Microbiol* 48 (1):253-267.

[143] Prigent-Combaret D, Lejeune P (1999) Monitoring gene expression in biofilms. Methods 310:56-79.

[144] Beloin C, Roux A, Ghigo J (2008) *Escherichia coli* biofilms. *Curr Top Microbiol Immunol* 322:249-289.

[145] Sutherland IW (2001) The biofilm matrix - an immobilized but dynamic microbial environment. *Trends Microbiol* 9:222-227.

[146] Prigent-Combaret C, Prensier G, Le Thi TT, Vidal OR, Ambert P, Lejeune P, Dorel C (2000) Developmental pathway for bioiflm formation in curli-producing *Escherichia coli* strains: role of flagella, curli and colanic acid. *J Bacteriol* 2:450-464.

[147] Zogaj X, Nimtz M, Rohde M, Bokranz W, Römling U (2001) The multicellular morphotypes of *Salmonella typhimurium* and *Escherichia*

coli produce cellulose as the second component of the extracellular matrix. *Mol Microbiol* 36 (6):1452-1463.
[148] Cookson AL, Cooley WA, Woodward MJ (2002) The role of type 1 and curli fimbriae of Shiga toxin-producing *Escherichia coli* in adherence to abiotic surfaces. *Int J Med Microbiol* 292:195-205.
[149] Schembri MA, Christiansen G, Klemm P (2001) FimH-mediated autoaggregation of *Escherichia coli. Mol Microbiol* 41:1419-1430.
[150] Römling U (2005) Characterization of the rdar morphotype, a multicellular behaviour in Enterobacteriaceae. *Cell Mol Life Sci* 62 (11):1234-1246.
[151] Barnhart MM, Chapman MR (2006) Curli biogenesis and function. Annu Rev Microbiol 60:131-147.
[152] Olsen A, Jonsson A, Normark S (1989) Fibronectin binding mediated by a novel class of surface organelles on *Escherichia coli. Nature* 338:652-655.
[153] Ben Nasr A, Olsén A, Sjöbring U, Müller-Esterl W, Björck L (1996) Assembly of human contact phase proteins and release of bradykinin at the surface of curli-expressing *Escherichia coli. Mol Microbiol* 20 (5):927-935.
[154] Gophna U, Barlev M, Seijffers R, Oelschlager TA, Hacker J, Ron EZ (2001) Curli fibers mediate internalization of *Escherichia coli* by eukaryotic cells. *Infect Immun* 69 (4):2659-2665.
[155] Bian A, Brauner A, Li Y, Normark S (2000) Expression of and cytokine activation by *Escherichia coli* curli fibers in human sepsis. *J Infect Dis* 181:602-612.
[156] Kai-Larsen Y, Lüthje P, Chromek M, Peters V, Wang X, Holm Å, Kádas L, Hedlund K, Johansson J, Chapman MR, Jacobson SH, Römling U, Agerberth B, Brauner A (2010) Uropathogenic *Escherichia coli* modulates immune responses and its curli fimbriae interact with the antimicrobial peptide LL-37. *PLoS Pathog* 6 (7):e1001010.
[157] Hammar M, Arnqvist A, Bian Z, Olsén A, Normark S (1995) Expression of two *csg* operons is required for production of fibronectin- and congo red-binding curli polymers in *Escherichia coli* K-12. *Mol Microbiol* 18 (4):661-670.
[158] Retegi A, Gabilondo N, Pena C, Zuluaga R, Castro C, Gana P, deleCaba K, Mondragon I (2010) Bacterial cellulose films with controlled microstructure-mechanical property relationships. *Cellulose* 17:661-669.

[159] Bokranz W, Wang X, Tschäpe H, Römling U (2005) Expression of cellulose and curli fimbriae by *Escherichia coli* isolated from the gastrointestinal tract. *J Med Microbiol* 54 (12):1171-1182.

[160] Da Re S, Ghigo J-M (2006) A CsgD-independent pathway for cellulose production and biofilm formation in *Escherichia coli. J Bacteriol* 188 (8):3073-3087.

[161] Gualdi L, Tagliabue L, Bertagnoli S, Ieranò T, De Castro C, Landini P (2008) Cellulose modulates biofilm formation by counteracting curli-mediated colonization of solid surfaces in *Escherichia coli. Microbiology* 154 (7):2017-2024.

[162] Zorraquino V, García B, Latasa C, Echeverz M, Toledo-Arana A, Valle J, Lasa I, Solano C (2012) Coordinated c-di-GMP repression of *Salmonella* motility through YcgR and cellulose. *J Bacteriol.*

[163] Wang X, Rochon M, Lamprokostopoulou A, Lünsdorf H, Nimtz M, Römling U (2006) Impact of biofilm matrix components on interaction of commensal *Escherichia coli* with the gastrointestinal cell line HT-29. *Cell Mol Life Sci* 63 (19):2352-2363.

[164] Lamprokostopoulou A, Monteiro C, Rhen M, Römling U (2010) Cyclic di-GMP signalling controls virulence properties of *Salmonella enterica* serovar *Typhimurium* at the mucosal lining. *Environ Microbiol* 12 (1):40-53.

[165] Norinder BS, Lüthje P, Yadav M, Kadas L, Fang H, Nord CE, Brauner A (2011) Cellulose and PapG are important for *Escherichia coli* causing recurrent urinary tract infection in women. *Infection* 39 (6):571-574.

[166] Rowe MC, Withers HL, Swift S (2010) Uropathogenic *Escherichia coli* forms biofilm aggregates under iron restriction that disperse upon the supply of iron. *FEMS Microbiol Lett* 307 (1):102-109.

[167] Solano C, García B, Valle J, Berasain C, Ghigo J-M, Gamazo C, Lasa I (2002) Genetic analysis of *Salmonella enteritidis* biofilm formation: critical role of cellulose. *Mol Microbiol* 43 (3):793-808.

[168] Mazur O, Zimmer J (2011) Apo- and cellopentaose-bound structures of the bacterial cellulose synthase subunit BcsZ. *J Biol Chem* 286 (20):17601-17606.

[169] Bhakdi S, Muhly M, Korom S, Schmidt G (1990) Effects of *Escherichia coli* hemolysin on human monocytes. *J Clin Invest* 85 (6):1746-1753.

[170] Cavalieri SJ, Bohach AA, Synder IS (1984) *Escherichia coli* α-hemolysin: characteristics and probable role in pathogenicity. *Microbiol Rev* 48:326-343.

[171] Konig B, Konig W, Scheffer J, Hacker J, Goebel W (1986) Role of *Escherichia coli* alpha-hemolysin and bacterial adherence in infection: requirement for release of inflammatory mediators from granulocytes and mast cells. *Infect Immun* 54:886-892.

[172] Keane WF, Welch R, Gekker G, Peterson PK (1987) Mechanism of *Escherichia coli* α-hemolysin-induced injury to isolated renal tubular cells. *Am J Pathol* 126 (350-357).

[173] Goebel W, Hedgpeth J (1982) Cloning and functional characterization of the plasmid-encoded hemolysin determinant of *Escherichia coli. J Bacteriol* 151:1290-1298.

[174] Hull SI, Hull RA, Minshew BH, Falkow S (1982) Genetics of hemolysin of *Escherichia coli.* J Bacteriol 151:1006-1012.

[175] Jorgensen SE, Short EC, Kurtz HJ, Mussen HK, Wu GK (1976) Studies on the origin of the α-haemolysin produced by *Escherichia coli. J Med Microbiol* 9:173-189.

[176] Jorgensen S, Mulcahy P, Wu G, Louis C (1983) Calcium accumulation in human and sheep erythrocytes that is induced by *Escherichia coli* hemolysin. *Toxicon* 21:717-727.

[177] Smith YC, Rasmussen SB, Grande KK, Conran RM, O'Brien AD (2008) Hemolysin of uropathogenic *Escherichia coli* evokes extensive shedding of teh uroepithelium and hemorrhage in bladder tissue within the first 24 hours after intraurethral inoculation of mice. *Infect Immun* 76 (7):2978-2990.

[178] Hilbert DW, Paulish-Miller TE, Tan CK, Carey AJ, Ulett GC, Mordechai E, Adelson ME, Gygax SE, Trama JP (2012) Clinical *Escherichia coli* isolates utilize alpha-hemolysin to inhibit *in vitro* epithelial cytokine production. *Microbes Infect* 14:628-638.

[179] Wilson KH, Blitchington RB (1996) Human colonic biota studied by ribosomal DNA sequence analysis. *Appl Environ Micro* 62:2273-2278.

[180] Siitonen A (1992) *Escherichia coli* in fecal flora of healthy adults: Serotypes, P and type 1C fimbriae, non-P manose-resistant adhesins, and hemolytic activity. *J Infect Dis* 166:1058-1065.

[181] Rippere-Lampe KE, O'Brien AD, Conran R, Lockman HA (2001) Mutation of the gene encoding cytotoxic necrotizing factor type 1 (cnf(1)) attenuates the virulence of uropathogenic *Escherichia coli. Infect Immun* 69:3954-3964.

[182] Trilfillis AL, Donnenberg MS, Cui X, Russell RG, Utsalo SJ, Mobley HL, Warren JW (1994) Binding to and killing of human renal epithelial cells by haemolytic P-fimbriated *E. coli. Kidney Int* 46:1083-1091.

[183] Wojnicz D (2007) Virulence factors of uropathogenic Escherichia coli strains isoalted from children with chronic pyelonephritis. *Adv Clin Exp Med* 16 (5):651-657.

[184] Tullus K, Jacobson SH, Katouli M, Brauner A (1991) Relative importance of eight virulence characteristics of pyelonephritogenic *Escherichia coli* strains assessed by multivarite statistical analysis. *J Urol 1*46 (4):1153-1155.

[185] Brauner A, Katouli M, Östenson CG (1995) P-fimbriation and haemolysin prodution are the most important virulence factors in diabetic patients with *Escherichia coli* bacteraemia: a multivariate statistical analysis of seven bacterial virulence factors. *J Infect* 31 (1):27-31.

[186] Hofman P, Le Negrate G, Mograbi B, Hofman V, Brest P, Alliana-Schmid A, Flatau G, Boquet P, Rossi B (2000) *Escherichia coli* cytotoxic necrotizing factor-1 (CNF-1) increases the adherence to epithelia and the oxidative burst of human polymorphonuclear leukocytes but decreases bacteria phagocytosis. *J Leukoc Biol* 68:522-528.

[187] Johnson DE, Drachenberg C, Lockatell CV, Island MD, Warren JW, Donnenberg MS (2000) The role of cytotoxic necrotizing factor-1 in colonization and tissue injury in a murine model of urinary tract infection. *FEMS Immunol Med Microbiol* 28:37-41.

[188] Rippere-Lampe KE, Lang M, Ceri H, Olson M, Lockman HA, O'Brien AD (2001) Cytotoxic necrotizing factor type 1-positive *Escherichia coli* causes increased inflammation and tissue damage to the prostate in a rat prostatitis model. *Infect Immun* 69:6515-6519.

[189] Brauner A, Katouli M, Tullus K, Jacobson SH (1990) Production of cytotoxic necrotizing factor, verocytotoxin and haemolysin by pyelonephritogenic *Escherichia coli. Eur J Clin Microbiol Infect Dis* 9:762-767.

[190] Johnson JR, Delavari P (2002) Concurrent fecal colonization with extraintestinal pathogenic *Escherichia coli* in a homosexual man with recurrent urinary tract infection and in his male sex partner. *Clin Infect Dis* 35:e65-68.

[191] Nemeth E, Rivera S, Gabayan V, Keller C, Taudorf S, Pedersen BK, Ganz T (2004) IL-6 mediated hypferremia of inflammation by inducing the synthesis of the iron regulatory hormone hepcidin. *J Clin Invest* 113 (9):1271-1276.

[192] Snyder JA, Haugenn BJ, Buckles EL, Lockatell CV, Johnson DE, Donnenberg MS, Welch RA, Mobley HLT (2004) Transcriptome of uropathogenic *Escherichia coli* during urinary tract infection. *Infect Immun* 72 (11):6373-6381.
[193] Rogers HJ (1973) Iron-binding catechols and virulence in *Escherichia coli*. *Infect Immun* 7 (3):445-456.
[194] Garcia EC, Brumbaugh AR, Mobley HLT (2011) Redundancy and specificity of *Escherichia coli* iron acquisition systems during urinary tract infection. *Infect Immun* 79 (3):1225-1235.
[195] Bauer RJ, Zhang L, Foxman B, Siitonen A, Jantunen ME, Saxen H, Marrs CF (2002) Molecular epidemiology of 3 putative virulence genes for *Escherichia coli* urinary tract infection - *usp*, *iha*, and $iroN_{E.\ coli}$. *J Infect Dis* 185:1521-1524.
[196] Fluckinger M, Haas H, Merschak P, Glasgow BJ, Redl B (2004) Human tear lipocalin exhibits antimicrobial activity by scavenging microbial siderophores. *Antimicrob Agents Chemother* 48 (9):3367-3372.
[197] Koczura R, Kaznowski A (2003) The Yersinia high-pathogenicity island and iron-uptake systems in clinical isolates of *Escherichia coli*. *J Med Microbiol* 52 (8):637-642.
[198] Caza M, Lépine F, Dozois CM (2011) Secretion, but not overall synthesis, of catecholate siderophores contributes to virulence of extraintestinal pathogenic *Escherichia coli*. *Mol Microbiol* 80 (1):266-282.
[199] Pi H, Jones SA, Mercer LE, Meador JP, Caughron JE, Jordon L, Newton SM, Conway T (2012) Role of catecholate siderophores in gram-negative bacterial colonization of the mouse gut. *PLoS One* 7 (11):e50020.
[200] Konopka K, Neilands JB (1984) Effect of serum albumin on siderophore-mediated utilization of transferrin iron. *Biochemistry* 23 (10):2122-2127.
[201] Herías MV, Midtvedt T, Hanson LÅ, Wold AE (1997) *Escherichia coli* K5 capsule expression enhances colonization of the large intestine in the gnotobiotic rat. *Infect Immun* 65 (2):531-536.
[202] Feldmann F, Sorsa LJ, Hildinger K, Schubert S (2007) The salmochelin siderophore receptor IroN contributes to invasion of urothelial cells by extraintestinal pathogenic *Escherichia coli* in vitro. *Infect Immun* 75 (6):3183-3187.
[203] Rabsch W, Voigt W, Reissbrodt R, Tsolis RM, Bäumler AJ (1999) *Salmonella typhimurium* IroN and FepA proteins mediate uptake of

enterobactin but differ in their specificity for other siderophores. *J Bacteriol* 181 (11):3610-3612.

[204] Watts RE, Totsika M, Challinor VL, Mabbett AN, Ulett GC, DeVoss JJ, Schembri MA (2012) Contribution of siderophore systems to growth and urinary tract colonization of asymptomatic bacteriuria *Escherichia coli*. *Infect Immun* 80 (1):333-344.

[205] Fischbach MA, Lin H, Zhou L, Yu Y, Abergel RJ, Liu DR, Raymond KN, Wanner BL, Strong RK, Walsh CT, Aderem A, Smith KD (2006) The pathogen-associated iroA gene cluster mediates bacterial evasion of lipocalin 2. *Proc Natl Acad Sci USA* 103 (44):16502-16507.

[206] Johnson JR, Stell AL (2000) Extended virulence genotypes of *Escherichia coli* strains from patients with urosepsis in relation to phylogeny and host compromise. *J Infect Dis* 181 (1):261-272.

[207] Henderson JP, Crowley JR, Pinkner JS, Walker JN, Tsukayama P, Stamm WE, Hooton TM, Hultgren SJ (2009) Quantitative metabolomics reveals an epigenetic blueprint for iron acquisition in uropathogenic *Escherichia coli*. *PLoS Pathog* 5 (2):e1000305.

[208] Hancock V, Ferrières L, Klemm P (2008) The ferric yersiniabactin uptake receptor FyuA is required for efficient biofilm formation by urinary tract infectious *Escherichia coli* in human urine. *Microbiology* 154 (1):167-175.

[209] Chaturvedi KS, Hung CS, Crowley JR, Stapleton AE, Henderson JP (2012) The siderophore yersiniabactin binds copper to protect pathogens during infection. *Nat Chem Biol* 8 (8):731-736.

[210] Valdebenito M, Crumbliss AL, Winkelmann G, Hantke K (2006) Environmental factors influence the production of enterobactin, salmochelin, aerobactin, and yersiniabactin in *Escherichia coli* strain Nissle 1917. *Int J Med Microbiol* 296:513-520.

[211] Vejborg RM, Hancock V, Schembri MA, Klemm P (2011) Comparative genomics of *Escherichia coli* strains causing urinary tract infections. *Appl Environ Microbiol* 77 (10):3268-3278.

[212] Marrs CF, Zhang L, Foxman B (2005) *Escherichia coli* mediated urinary tract infections: are there distinct uropathogenic *E. coli* (UPEC) pathotypes? *FEMS Microbiol Lett* 252:183-190.

[213] Burns SM, Hull SI (1999) Loss of resistance to ingestion and phagocytic killing by O− and K− mutants of a uropathogenic *Escherichia coli* O75:K5 strain. *Infect Immun* 67 (8):3757-3762.

[214] Hughes CL, Phillips R, Roberts AP (1982) Serum resistance among *Escherichia coli* strains causing urinary tract infection in relation to O

type and the carriage of haemolysin, colicin, and antibiotic resistance determinants. *Infect Immun* 40:265-272.

[215] Llobet E, Tomas J, Bengoechea J (2008) Capsule polysaccharide is a bacterial decoy for antimicrobial peptides. *Microbiology* 154:3877-3886.

[216] Schembri MA, Dalsgaard D, Klemm P (2004) Capsule shields the function of short bacterial adhesins. *J Bacteriol* 186 (5):1249-1257.

[217] Valle J, Da Re S, Henry N, Fontaine T, Balestrino D, Latour-Lambert P, Ghigo J-M (2006) Broad-spectrum biofilm inhibition by a secreted bacterial polysaccharide. *Proc Natl Acad Sci USA* 103 (33):12558-12563.

[218] Marrs CF, Zhang L, Tallman P, Manning SD, Somsel P, Raz P, Colodner R, Jantunen ME, Siitonen A, Saxen H, Foxman B (2002) Variations in 10 putative uropathogen virulence genes among urinary, faecal and peri-urethral *Escherichia coli*. *J Med Microbiol* 51:138-142.

[219] Öhman L, Tullus K, Katouli M, Burman L, Stendahl O (1995) Correlation between susceptibility of infants to infection and interaction with neutrophils of *Escherichia coli* strains causing neonatal and infantile septicemia. *J Infect Dis* 171:128-133.

[220] Mulder CJ, Van Alphen L, Zanen HC (1984) Neonatal meningitis caused by *Escherichia coli* in The Netherlands. *J Infect Dis* 150:935-940.

[221] Bingen-Bidois M, Clermont O, Bonacorsi S, Terki M, Brahimi N, Loukil C, Barraud D, Bingen E (2002) Phylogenetic analysis and prevalence or urosepsis strains of *Escherichia coli* bearing pathogenicity island-like domains. *Infect Immun* 70 (6):3216-3226.

[222] Troy FA (1992) Polysialylation: from bacteria to brains. *Glycobiology* 2:5-23.

[223] Anderson G, Goller C, Justice S, Hultgren SJ, Seed P (2010) Polysaccharide capsule and sialic acid-mediated regulation promote biofilm-like intracellular bacterial communities during cystitis. *Infect Immun* 78:963-975.

[224] Ikäheimo R, Siitonen A, Kärkkäinen U, Kuosmanen P, Mäkelä PH (1993) Characteristics of *Escherichia coli* in acute community-acquired cystitis of adult women. *Scand J Infect Dis* 25 (6):705-712.

[225] Montenegro M, Bitter-Suermann D, Timmis JK, Aguero M, Cabello F, Sanyal S, Timmis K (1985) *tra*T gene sequences, serum resistance and pathogenicity-related factors in clinical isolates of *Escherichia coli* and other gram-negative bacteria. *J Gen Microbiol* 131:1511-1521.

[226] Wang L, Rothemund D, Curd H, Reeves PR (2003) Species-wide variation in the *Escherichia coli* flagellin (H-antigen) gene. *J Bacteriol* 185 (9):2936-2943.
[227] Johnson J, Orskov I, Orskov F, Goulet P, Picard B, Moseley S, Roberts P, Stamm W (1994) O, K, and H antigens predict virulence factors, carboxyesterase B pattern, antimicrobial ressitance and host compromise among *Escherichia coli* strains causing urosepsis. *J Infect Dis* 169:119-126.
[228] Ørskov F, Ørskov I (1992) Escherichia coli serotyping and disease in man and animals. *Can J Microbiol* 38:7.
[229] Clermont O, Johnson JR, Menard M, Denamur E (2007) Determination of *Escherichia coli* O types by allele-specific polymerase chain reaction: application to the O types involved in human septicemia. *Diagn Microbiol Infect Dis* 57:129-136.
[230] Lin A, Sultan O, Lau HK, Wong E, Hartman G, Lauzon C (2011) O serogroup specific real time PCR assays for the detection and identification of nine clinically relevant non-O157 STECs. *Food Microbiol* 28:478-483.
[231] Ejrnaes K, Sandvang D, Lundgren B, Ferry S, Holm S, Monsen T, Lundholm R, Frimodt-Møller N (2006) Pulsed-field gel electrophoresis typing of *Escherichia coli* strains from samples collected before and after pivmecillinam or placebo treatment of uncomplicated community-acquired urinary tract infection in women. *J Clin Microbiol* 44 (5):1776-1781.
[232] Skjøt-Rasmussen L, Hammerum AM, Jakobsen L, Lester CH, Larsen P, Frimodt-Møller N (2011) Persisting clones of *Escherichia coli* isolates from recurrent urinary tract infection in men and women. *J Med Microbiol* 60 (4):550-554.
[233] Hunstad DA, Justice SS (2010) Intracellular lifestyles and Iimmune evasion strategies of uropathogenic *Escherichia coli. Ann Rev Microbiol* 64 (1):203-221.
[234] Goller C, Seed P (2010) Revisiting the *Escherichia coli* polysaccharide capsule as a virulence factor during urinary tract infection: Contribution to intracellular biofilm development. *Virulence* 1:333-337.
[235] Maki N, Gestwicki JE, Lake EM, Kiessling LL, Adler J (2000) Motility and chemotaxis of filamentous cells of *Escherichia coli. J Bacteriol* 182 (15):4337-4342.

[236] Justice SS, Hunstad DA, Seed PC, Hultgren SJ (2006) Filamentation by *Escherichia coli* subverts innate defenses during urinary tract infection. *Proc Natl Acad Sci USA* 103 (52):19884-19889.

[237] Rosen DA, Hooton TM, Stamm WE, Humphrey PA, Hultgren SJ (2007) Detection of intracellular bacterial communities in human urinary tract infection. *PLoS Med* 4 (12):e329.

[238] Johnson JR, Roberts PL, Stamm WE (1987) P fimbriae and other virulence factors in *Escherichia coli* urosepsis: association with patients' characteristics. *J Infect Dis* 156 (1):225-229.

[239] Gunther IV NW, Lockatell V, Johnson DE, Mobley HLT (2001) In vivo dynamics of type 1 fimbria regulation in uropathogenic *Escherichia coli* during experimental urinary tract infection. *Infect Immun* 69 (5):2838-2846.

[240] Holden NJ, Uhlin BE, Gally DL (2001) PapB paralogues and their effect on the phase variation of type 1 fimbriae in *Escherichia coli. Mol Microbiol* 42 (2):319-330.

[241] Xia Y, Gally D, Forsmann-Semb K, Uhlin BE (2000) Regulatory cross-talk between adhesin operons in *Escherichia coli:* inhibition of type 1 fimbriae expression by the PapB protein. *EMBO J* 19:1450-1457.

[242] Svanborg-Eden C, Hansson HA (1978) *Escherichia coli* pili as possible mediators of attachment to human urinary tract epithelial cells. *Infect Immun* 21:229-237.

[243] Korhonen TK, Virkola R, Holthofer H (1986) Localization of binding sites for purified *Escherichia coli* P fimbriae in the human kidney. *Infect Immun* 54:328-332.

[244] Elo J, Tallgren LG, Vaisanen V, Korhonen TK, Svenson SB, Makela PH (1985) Association of P and other fimbriae with clinical pyelonephritis in children. *Scand J Urol Nephrol* 19:281-284.

[245] Oelschlaeger TA, Dobrindt U, Hacker J (2002) Pathogenicity islands of uropathogenic *E. coli* and the evolution of virulence. *Int J of Antmicrobial Agents* 19:517-521.

[246] Diard M, Garry L, Selva M, Mosser T, Denamur E, Matic I (2010) Pathogenicity-associated islands in extraintestinal pathogenic *Escherichia coli* are fitness elements inolved in intestinal colonization. *J Bacteriol* 192 (19):4885-4893.

[247] Frost LS, Leplae R, Summers AO, Toussaint A (2005) Mobile genetic elements: the agents of open source evolution. *Nat Rev Microbiol* 3 (722-732).

[248] Couturier M, Bex F, Bergquist P, Maas W (1988) Identification and classficiation of bacterial plasmids. *Microbiol Rev* 52:375-395.

[249] Johnson TJ, Nolan LK (2009) Pathogenomics of the virulence plasmids of *Escherichia coli*. Microbiol *Mol Biol Rev* 73 (4):750-774.

[250] Carattoli A, Bertini A, Villa L, Falbo V, Hopkins KL, EJ T (2005) Identification of plasmids by PCR-based replicon typing. *J Microbiol Methods* 63 (3):219-228.

[251] Johnson JR, Kuskowsky MA, Gajewski A, Sahm DF, Karlowsky JA (2004) Virulence characteristics and phylogenetic background of multidrug-resistant and antimicrobial-susceptible clinical isolates of Escherichia coli from across the United States, 2000-2001. *J Infect Dis* 190:1739-1744.

[252] Oswald E, Sugai M, Labigne A, Wu HC, Fiorentini C, Boquet P, O'Brien AD (1994) Cytotoxic necrotizing factor type 2 produced by virulent *Escherichia coli* modified the small GTP-binding proteins Rho involved in assembly of actin stress fibers. *Proc Natl Acad Sci USA* 91:3814-3818.

[253] Rijavec M, Erjavec MS, Avguštin JA, Reissbrodt R, Fruth A, Križan-Hergouth V, Žgur-Bertok D (2006) High prevalence of multidrug resistance and random distribution of mobile genetic elements among uropathogenic *Escherichia coli* (UPEC) of the four major phylogenetic groups. *Curr Microbiol* 53:158-162.

[254] Dobrindt U, Janke B, Piechaczek K, Nagy G, Ziebuhr W, Fischer G, Schierhorn A, Hecker M, Blum-Oehler G, Hacker J (2000) Toxin genes on pathogenicity islands: impact for microbial evolution. *Int J Med Microbiol* 290 (4-5):307-311.

[255] Wiles TJ, Kulesus RR, Mulvey MA (2008) Origins and virulence mechanisms of uropathogenic *Escherichia coli*. *Exp Mol Pathol* 85:11-19.

[256] Van Den Bosch JF, deGraaff J, MacLaren DM (1979) Virulence of *Escherichia coli* in experimental hematogenous pyelonephritis in mice. *Infect Immun* 25 (1):68-74.

[257] Blanco M, Blanco JE, Alonso MP, Blanco J (1996) Virulence factors and O groups of *Escherichia coli* isolates from patients with acute pyelonephritis, cystitis and asymptomatic bacteriuria. *Eur J Epidemiol* 12:191-198.

[258] Russo TA, Stapleton A, Wenderoth S, Hooton TM, Stamm W (1995) Chromosomal restriction fragment length polymorphism analysis of

Escherichia coli strains causing recurrent urinary tract infections in young women. *J Infect Dis* 172:440-445.

[259] Foxman B (2010) The epidemiology of urinary tract infection. *Nat Rev Urol* 7 (12):653-660.

[260] Manges AR, Johnson JR, Foxman B, O'Bryan TT, Fullerton KE, Riley LW (2001) Widespread distribution of urinary tract infections caused by a multidrug-resistant *Escherichia coli* clonal group. *N Engl J Med* 345 (14):1007-1013.

[261] Phillips I, Eykyn S, King A, Gransden WR, Rowe B, Frost JA, Gross RJ (1988) Epidemic multiresistant *Escherichia coli* infection in West Lambeth Health District. *Lancet* 7 (1):1038-1041.

[262] Olesen B, Kolmos HJ, Orskov F, Orskov I (1994) Cluster of multiresistant *Escherichia coli* O78:H10 in greater Copenhagen. *Scand J Infect Dis* 26 (4):406-410.

[263] Foxman B, Manning SD, Tallman P, Bauer R, Zhang L, Koopman S, Gillespie B, Sobel JD, Marrs CF (2002) Uropathogenic *Escherichia coli* are more likely than commensal *E. coli* to be shared between heterosexual sex partners. *Am J Epidemiol* 156:1133-1140.

[264] Foxman B, Zhang L, Tallman P, Andree BC, Geiger AM, Koopman JS, Gillespie BW, Palin KA, Sobel JD (1997) Transmission of uropathogens between sex partners. *J Infect Dis* 175:989-992.

[265] Johnson JR, Owens K, Gajewski A, Clabots C (2008) *Escherichia coli* colonization patterns among human household members and pets, with attention to acute urinary tract infection. *J Infect Dis* 197:218-224.

[266] Nicolas-Chanoine M, Blanco J, Leflon-Guibout V, Demarty R, Alonso MP, Canica MM, Park Y, Lavigne J (2008) Intercontinental emergence of *Escherichia coli* clone O25:H4-ST131 producing CTX-M-15. *J Antimicrob Chemother* 61:273-281.

[267] Coque TM, Novais A, Carattoli A, Poirel L, Pitout J, Peixe L, Baquero F, Canton R, Nordmann P (2008) Dissemination of clonally related *Escherichia coli* strains expressing extended-spectrum ß-lactamase CTX-M-15. *Emerg Infect Dis* 14 (2):195-200.

[268] Lau SH, Reddy S, Cheesbrough J, Bolton FJ, Willshaw G, Cheasty T, Fox AJ, Upton M (2008) Major uropathogenic *Escherichia coli* strain isolated in the northwest of England identified by multilocus sequence typing. *J Clin Microbiol* 46 (3):1076-1080.

[269] Johnson JR, Johnston B, Clabots C, Kuskowski MA, Pendyala S, DebRoy C, Nowicki B, Rice J (2010) *Escherichia coli* sequence type ST131 as an emerging fluoroquinolone-resistant uropathogen among

renal transplant recipients. *Antimicrob Agents Chemother* 54 (1):546-550.

[270] Johnson JR, Miller S, Johnston B, Clabots C, DebRoy C (2009) Sharing of *Escherichia coli* sequence type ST131 and other multidrug-resistant and urovirulent *E. coli* strains among dogs and cats within a household. *J Clin Microbiol* 47 (11):3721-3725.

[271] Ewers C, Grobbel M, Stamm I, Kopp PA, Diehl I, Semmler T, Fruth A, Beutlich J, Guerra B, Wieler LH, Guenther S (2010) Emergence of human pandemic O25:H4-ST131 CTX-M-15 extended-spectrum-ß-lactamase-producing *Escherichia coli* among companion animals. *J Antimicrob Chemother* 65:651-660.

[272] Rogers BA, Sidjabat HE, Paterson DL (2010) Escherichia coli O25b-ST131: a pandemic, multiresistant, community-associated strain. *J Antimicrob Chemother.*

[273] Moreno E, Andreu A, Pérez T, Sabaté M, Johnson JR, Prats G (2006) Relationship between *Escherichia coli* strains causing urinary tract infection in women and the dominant faecal flora of the same hosts. *Epidemiol Infect* 134:1015-1023.

[274] Frömmel U, Lehmann W, Rödiger S, Böhm A, Nitschke J, Weinreich J, Groß J, Roggenbuck D, Zinke O, Ansorge H, Vogel S, Klemm P, Wex T, Schröder C, Wieler LH, Schierack P (2013) Adhesion of human and animal *Escherichia coli* strains in association with their virulence-associated genes and phylogenetic origins. *Appl Environ Microbiol* 79 (19):5814-5829.

[275] Stamey TA (1973) The role of introital enterobacteria in recurrent urinary infections. *J Urol* 109:467-472.

[276] Stamey TA, Timothy M, Millar M, Mihara G (1971) Recurrent urinary infections in adult women. The role of introital enterobacteria. *Calif Med* 115:1-19.

[277] Schlager T, Hendley J, Lohr J, Whittam T (1993) Effect of periurethral colonization on the risk of urinary tract infection in healthy girls after their first urinary tract infection. *Pediatr Infect Dis J* 12:988-993.

[278] Hung CS, Dodson KW, Hultgren SJ (2009) A murine model of urinary tract infection. *Nat Protoc* 4:1230-1243.

[279] Davies CM, Long JA, Donald M, Ashbolt NJ (1995) Survival of fecal microorganisms in marine and freshwater sediments. *Appl Environ Microbiol* 61 (5):1888-1896.

[280] Fujioka RS, Hashimoto HH, Siwak EB, Young RH (1981) Effect of sunlight on survival of indicator bacteria in seawater. *Appl Environ Microbiol* 41q (3):690-696.

[281] Anastasi EM, Matthews B, Stratton HM, Katouli M (2012) Pathogenic *Escherichia coli* found in sewage treatment plants and environmental waters. *Appl Environ Microbiol* 78 (16):5536-5541.

[282] Johnson JR, Kuskowski MA, Smith K, O'Bryan TT, Tatini S (2005) Antimicrobial-resistant and extraintestinal pathogenic *Escherichia coli* in retail foods. *J Infect Dis* 191 (7):1040-1049.

[283] Escobar-Páramo P, Le Menac'h A, Le Gall T, Amorin C, Gouriou S, Picard B, Skurnik D, Denamur E (2006) Identification of forces shaping the commensal *Escherichia coli* genetic structure by comparing animal and human isolates. *Environ Microbiol* 8 (11):1975-1984.

[284] Armand-Lefevre L, Ruimy R, Andremont A (2005) Clonal comparison of *Staphylococcus aureus* isolate from healthy pig farmers, human controls, and pigs. *Emerg Infect Dis* 11 (5):711-714.

In: Urinary Tract Infections
Editor: Kristen E. Murrell

ISBN: 978-1-63117-180-2

Chapter 4

Treatment for Urinary Tract Infections due to Multidrug-Resistant Bacteria

Thana Khawcharoenporn,[1*] and Kamaljit Singh,[2]

[1]Division of Infectious Diseases, Faculty of Medicine, Thammasat University, Pathumthani, Thailand

[2]Section of Infectious Diseases, Rush University Medical Center, Chicago, IL, US

Abstract

Inappropriate use of antibiotics together with evolving resistance of bacteria has increased the prevalence of infections due to multidrug-resistant (MDR) bacteria worldwide over the past few decades. Urinary tract infections are amongst the most common infectious diseases affected by the increasing burden of antibiotic resistance. Selection of appropriate empiric and definite antibiotic therapy for urinary tract infection (UTI) has become more challenging for healthcare providers resulting in delay in appropriate therapy. Several factors need to be taken

* Corresponding author: Thana Khawcharoenporn, MD, MSc, Division of Infectious Diseases, Faculty of Medicine, Thammasat University, Pathumthani, Thailand 12120, E-mail: thanak30@yahoo.com.

into account for antibiotic selection. These include patient's characteristics, history of prior UTI treatment, previous antibiotic exposure and local antibiotic resistance pattern. Some of the uropathogenic MDR bacteria that are threats for healthcare system include gram-positive MDR bacteria, such as methicillin-resistant *Staphylococcus aureus* and vancomycin-resistant enterococci and gram-negative MDR bacteria, such as the Enterobacteriaceae, *Pseudomonas aeruginosa* and *Acinetobacter baumannii*. Urinary tract infections due to these organisms require early appropriate antibiotic treatment to prevent morbidity and mortality. In some cases, novel methods of antibiotic administration including combination therapy and prolonged infusion therapy may be required. In complicated cases, combined surgical interventions are needed along with antibiotic therapy. In addition, infection control measures are necessary to prevent further transmission of these MDR bacteria between patients and within a hospital. This chapter reviews the epidemiology of MDR bacteria, appropriate empiric and definite treatments and adjunctive measures and strategies to manage UTIs caused by the MDR bacteria.

Introduction

Infections due to drug-resistant bacteria have emerged as major public threats worldwide for the past few decades. The rates of antibiotic resistance among gram-positive and gram-negative bacteria have increased and vary depending on geographic areas. The major factor for development of antibiotic resistance is the widespread and inappropriate use of antibiotics. This exerts pressure to select naturally mutant resistant bacterial strains or to evolve and acquire antibiotic resistance in order to survive. Inappropriate use of antibiotics may include empiric antibiotic treatment without indication, use of antibiotics that are not active or partially active against bacteria, non-targeted use of broad-spectrum antibiotics and use of inadequate dose and duration of antibiotics. Drug-resistant bacteria-associated infections are of global health concern given their associations with limited treatment options, low treatment efficacy, significant patient morbidity and mortality, utilization of limited resources and increase in length of hospital stay and cost. [1-4]

Urinary tract infections (UTIs) are one of the most common infections among patients in both community and healthcare settings. The most common causative uropathogens are the Enterobacteriaceae which generally colonize the gastrointestinal tracts. Gram-positive bacteria are less common pathogens and usually associated with complicated infections. Among community-associated UTIs, empiric treatment should target the Enterobacteriaceae especially *Escherichia coli* while healthcare-associated UTIs require empiric treatment that is active against nosocomial pathogens, such as *Pseudomonas aeruginosa, Acinetobacter spp., Staphylococcus aureus* and Enterococci in addition to the Enterobacteriaceae. Empiric therapy is selected based on local resistance patterns, drug availability, and antibiotic intolerance/allergy history of treated patients. [5,6] Choosing empiric therapy for UTIs has become more challenging in the era of increasing antibiotic resistance as commonly used antibiotics, such as trimethoprim-sulfamethoxazole (TMP-SMX) and fluoroquinolones may no longer be appropriate. The epidemiology, appropriate antibiotic treatment, adjunctive measures and strategies to manage drug-resistant bacterial UTIs are reviewed in this chapter.

Definitions

Types of Urinary Tract Infection

There are many types of UTIs. For clinical management purposes, they are usually categorized into lower UTIs and upper UTIs or uncomplicated UTIs and complicated UTIs. Lower UTIs include infections of the urinary tract from bladder to the urethra opening, such as cystitis, urethritis, and prostatitis while upper UTIs are infections of the urinary tract above the bladder to kidneys and tissues around the kidneys, such as pyelonephritis, renal abscess, perinephric abscess, bacteremic UTIs and urosepsis. Complicated UTIs are defined as UTIs occurring in a patient with a structural or functional abnormality of the genitourinary tract including obstruction, instrumentation, impaired voiding, metabolic abnormalities such as diabetes, immunocompromized status, UTIs in male, UTIs caused by nosocomial or antibiotic-resistant pathogens and UTIs associated with suppurative complications, such as renal or perirenal abscesses, and metastatic infections including bone and joint infection or endocarditis. [7,8] Urinary tract infections without these features are considered uncomplicated UTIs. The purposes of such UTI categorization schemes are mainly to guide duration and type of antibiotic treatment and to determine whether further intervention and closer monitoring are needed for patient management. Generally, complicated UTIs are associated with increased risk for drug-resistant bacteria infections which are the focus of the next section.

Multidrug Resistance

Definitions for types of bacterial multidrug resistance have been published by a group of international experts in a joint initiative by the European Centre for Disease Prevention and Control and the Centers for Disease Control and Prevention. [9] Three types of multidrug resistance are defined; multidrug-resistance (MDR), extensively drug-resistance (XDR) and pandrug resistance (PDR). MDR bacteria are bacteria that are non-susceptible to at least one agent in 3 or more categories of antibiotics used against these bacteria while XDR bacteria are non-susceptible to at least one agent in all except 2 or less categories of antibiotics used against these bacteria. Bacteria with PDR are non-susceptible to all agents in all categories of antibiotics used against these bacteria. PDR bacteria are subsets of XDR bacteria and both PDR and XDR bacteria are subsets of MDR bacteria. Examples of *E. coli* isolates' antibiotic susceptibility profiles consistent with non-MDR, MDR, XDR and PDR isolates are shown in Table 1.

Epidemiology

Important MDR bacteria causing UTIs can be divided into 2 groups; Gram-positive bacteria and Gram-negative bacteria.

Gram-Positive Bacteria

Enterococcus spp. and *Staphylococcus aureus*

Enterococcus spp. and Staphylococcus aureus account for the majority of UTIs due to Gram-positive bacteria. Results from the North American Urinary Tract Infection Collaborative Alliance (NAUTICA) in 2005 indicated that 6.6% and 2.2% of outpatient urinary isolates were *Enterococcus spp.* and *Staphylococcus aureus*, respectively. [10] Among healthcare-associated UTIs, mainly catheter-associated UTIs (CA-UTI) reported by the National Healthcare Safety Network (NHSN) at the Centers for Disease Control and Prevention, 10.3% were caused by *Enterococcus spp.* and 2.1% were caused by *Staphylococcus* aureus. [11] MDR *Enterococcus spp.* are usually resistance to penicillin, ampicillin, piperacillin-tazobactam, levofloxacin, nitrofuratoin and vancomycin. These strains are most commonly known as vancomycin-resistant *Enterococcus spp.* (VRE). In the NHSN data, 83% of *Enterococcus faecium*-associated CA-UTIs were vancomycin-resistant while 8% of *Enterococcus faecalis*-associated CA-UTIs were vancomycin-resistant. [11]

Table 1. Examples of *Escherichia coli* isolates' antibiotic susceptibility profiles consistent with non-MDR, MDR, XDR and PDR isolates

Antibiotic category	Antibiotic name	Susceptibility			
		Non-MDR	MDR	XDR	PDR
Penicillins	Penicllin	R	R	R	R
	Ampicillin	R	R	R	R
	Amoxicillin-clavulanate	S	S	R	R
	Ampicillin-sulbactam	S	S	R	R
	Piperacillin-tazobactam	S	S	R	R
Cephalosporins	Cefazolin	S	R	R	R
	Cefuroxime	S	R	R	R
	Ceftriaxone	S	R	R	R
	Ceftazidime	S	R	R	R

Table 1. (Continued)

Antibiotic category	Antibiotic name	Susceptibility			
		Non-MDR	MDR	XDR	PDR
	Cefepime	S	R	R	R
Carbapenems	Ertapenem	S	S	S	R
	Imipenem	S	S	S	R
	Meropenem	S	S	S	R
	Doripenem	S	S	S	R
Fluoroquinolones	Ciprofloxacin	S	R	R	R
	Levofloxacin	S	R	R	R
Aminoglycosides	Gentamicin	S	S	S	R
	Amikacin	S	S	S	R
Sulfonamides	Trimethoprim-sulfamethoxazole	R	R	R	R
Nitrofurantoin	Nitrofurantoin	S	S	R	R

NOTE: MDR = multidrug-resistant; XDR = extensively drug-resistant; PDR = pandrug-resistant; S = susceptible; R = resistant.

Table 2. Endemic areas and risk factors for acquisition of multidrug-resistant Gram-positive bacteria

Bacteria	Endemic areas	Risk factors
Vancomycin-resistant enterococci (VRE)	Worldwide, mainly reported from the US [101-107]	Prior vancomycin use [101,103,105,107,108] Prior aminoglycoside use within 30 days [104] Prior carbapenem use within 30 days [104] Prior fluoroquinolone use [105,106] Prior 3rd generation cephalosporin use [106,107] Prior metronidazole use [106] Previous colonization with VRE [102] Admission from long-term care facility [103] Being placed in a VRE-contaminated room [105]
Methicillin-resistant *Staphylococcus aureus* (MRSA)	Healthcare-associated MRSA - Worldwide	Prior fluoroquinolone use [13,14] Prior cephalosporin use [14] HIV infection [109,110] Being on hemodialysis [15] Prolonged hospitalization [16,17] Receipt of intensive care [16,17] Presence of indwelling medical device [16,17] Previous colonization with MRSA [18] Proximity to others with MRSA colonization/infection [16,17]
	Community-associated MRSA – Worldwide, mainly in the US, Europe, Australia and some countries in Asia, such as Sri Lanka, Taiwan, Vietnam, the Philippines and Korea [12]	Native communities (American/Indian) [20] Sports teams [21] Men who have sex with men [19] Prison inmates [22] Military personnel [22] Close contact with person colonized with MRSA [23]

Several factors and patient's characteristics are identified as risk factors associated with VRE infections as shown in Table 2. Of note, prior use of several antibiotics, prior colonization with VRE and being in an environment contaminated with VRE are important risks. MDR *Staphylococcus aureus* are usually referred to methicillin-resistant *Staphylococcus aureus* (MRSA) which can be further divided into 2 groups; healthcare-associated MRSA (HA-MRSA) and community-associated MRSA (CA-MRSA). These 2 groups are different in terms of genetic and molecular characteristics, virulence factors, prerequisite infected sites and susceptibility to antibiotics. HA-MRSA is usually resistant to all beta-lactam antibiotics, such as penicillins, cephalosporins and carbapenems, and non-beta-lactam antibiotics, such as fluoroquinolones, TMP-SMX, clindamycin and tetracyclines while CA-MRSA is resistant to all beta-lactam antibiotics but is usually susceptible to non-beta-lactam antibiotics, especially TMP-SMX, doxycycline, and clindamycin. In the NHSN data, 50% of *Staphylococcus aureus*-associated CA-UTIs were MRSA. [11] While infections due to HA-MRSA are common in several regions, CA-MRSA associated infections are endemic in some parts of the world i.e., the US, Europe and Australia. There are increasing number of CA-MRSA associated infections in Asia, especially in Sri Lanka, Taiwan, Vietnam, the Philippines and Korea. [12] Endemic areas and risk factors for acquisitions of both HA-MRSA and CA-MRSA are shown in Table 2. UTIs caused by MRSA are usually results of hematogenous spread from invasive MRSA infections. Risk factors for HA-MRSA associated infections include prior antibiotic use, presence of indwelling medical devices, receipt of intensive care and prolonged hospitalization. [13-18] CA-MRSA associated infections are associated with different risks which include being in native communities, overcrowding, playing contact sports, and being men who have sex with men, prison inmates, and military personnel. [19-23]

Gram-Negative Bacteria

Extended-Spectrum Beta-Lactamase (ESBL) Producing Enterobacteriaceae

The Enterobacteriaceae are the most common pathogens causing UTIs. ESBL production are most commonly seen in *E. coli, Klebsiella spp.* and *Proteus mirabilis* and these organisms can be regarded as MDR Enterobacteriaceae. In the NHSN data, 27% of *Klebsiella spp.* and 12% of *E. coli* were ESBL producers among the CA-UTI cases. [11] A recent study from the US revealed that ESBL producing Enterobacteriaceae accounted for 24% of all MDR Enterobacteriaceae isolates causing UTIs. [24] In the Asia-Pacific region where ESBL-producing Enterobacteriaceae are endemic, 37% of Enterobacteriaceae isolated from patients with upper UTIs were ESBL-producers. [25]

Table 3. Endemic areas and risk factors for acquisition of multidrug-resistant Gram-negative bacteria

Bacteria	Endemic areas	Risk factors
ESBL-producing Enterobacteriaceae	Worldwide	Prolonged hospital stay [28,29] Prolonged intensive care unit stay [28,29] Presence of central venous or arterial catheter [28,29] Presence of urinary catheter [28,29] Presence of gastrostomy or jejunostomy tube [28,29] Ventilatory assistance [28,29] Emergency abdominal surgery [28,29] Receipt of hemodialysis [28] Prior use of any antibiotics (especially, 2nd or 3rd generation cephalosporins) [28-30] Prior residence in a long-term care facility [28,29] Severity of illness [28,29]
Carbapenem-resistant Enterobacteriaceae (CRE)	USA (CRE, KPC) [34-36] Canada (CRE, NDM-1) [111] Greece [33] United Kingdom (NDM-1) [32] India (CRE, NDM-1) [32]	Prior carbapenem, 3rd and 4th generation cephalosporin use [112] Prior fluoroquinolone use [113] Prior glycopeptide use [114] Prior metronidazole use [115] Exposure to healthcare in endemic countries [32] Recent organ or stem cell transplantation [112] Receipt of mechanical ventilation [112] Prolonged hospital stay [112] Higher APACHE II score [116] Presence of catheter [115]

Table 3. (Continued)

Bacteria	Endemic areas	Risk factors
Carbapenem-resistant *Pseudomonas aeruginosa* (CRP)	Brazil [37] Thailand [38] India [39] South Korea [40,41] USA [42,43] European countries [44]	Prior group 2 carbapenem use [41,43] Prior piperacillin-tazobactam use [41,43] Prior fluoroquinolone use [41,117] Prior aminoglycoside use [43] Prior vancomycin use [41,43] Presence of urinary catheter [118] Previous *P. aeruginosa* colonization/infection [119] Receipt of mechanical ventilation [120] Prolonged hospital stay [119] Previous hospitalization [120] High APACHE II score [121] Presence of CRP in the same unit [119]
Carbapenem-resistant *Acinetobacter baumannii* (CRA)	Australia [45] Brazil [46] Canada [47] Greece [48] South Korea [49] Spain [50] Taiwan [51] Thailand [52]	Prior group 2 carbapenem use [51] Prior aminopenicillin use [122] Prolonged hospital stay [51] Prior *A. baumannii* colonization [51] Presence of catheter [50] High APACHE II score [123] Recent surgery [50] High prevalence of CRA-colonized patients in the same unit [124]

NOTE: APACHE = acute physiology and chronic health evaluation; KPC = *Klebsiella pneumoniae* carbapenemase; NDM = New Delhi metallo-betalactamase.

There have been increasing reports of community-associated ESBL-producing Enterobacteriaceae UTIs in the past decade. The prevalence of this type of UTI was reported to be 30% in Latin America [26] and 27% in India. [27] ESBL-producing Enterobacteriaceae are generally resistant to penicillins, 1st to 4th generation cephalosporins and aztreonam. These organisms may also be resistant to TMP-SMX, fluoroquinolones or aminoglycosides. Important risk factors for ESBL-producing Enterobacteriaceae UTIs are summarized in Table 3. Theses mainly include prolonged hospital stay, presence of devices, prior use of any antibiotics, especially 2nd and 3rd generation cephalosporins, severity of illness and being on hemodialysis. [28-30]

Carbapenem-Resistant Enterobacteriaceae (CRE)

There have been increasing reports of CRE associated infections in many regions of the world during the past decade. [31] The three countries with the highest incidences of CRE infections, mainly reported from tertiary-care centers, were Greece (20–50%), India (4–24%) and the USA (4–11%). [32-36] Further investigations revealed that some of these CRE strains were *Klebsiella pneumoniae* carbapenemases (KPCs) and New Delhi metallo-β-lactamase (NDM)-1-producing Enterobacteriaceae. CREs are generally resistant to all beta-lactam antibiotics including penicillins, cephalosporins and carbapenems, TMP-SMX, fluoroquinolones and nitrofurantoin. The remaining antibiotics that these organisms may be susceptible to are aminoglycosides, colistin, tigecycline and fosfomycin. Endemic areas for specific types of CREs and risk factors for acquisition of CRE-associated infections are summarized in Table 3. Prior use of antibiotics especially carbapenems, 3rd and 4th generation cephalosporins and fluoroquinolones is an important risk. In addition, exposures to healthcare in countries where CREs are endemic increase risk of CRE acquisition, especially for NDM-1-producing Enterobacteriaceae.

Multidrug-Resistant Pseudomonas aeruginosa

Pseudomonas aeruginosa is one of the most common pathogens causing healthcare-associated infections worldwide. MDR *P. aeruginosa* isolates are resistant to at least 1 drug in 3 of the 5 following antibiotic classes including antipseudomonal penicillins, antipseudomonal cephalosporins, fluoroquinolones, aminoglycosides and carbapenems. Data from NHSN indicated that 14% of *P. aeruginosa* isolates causing CA-UTI were MDR. [11] Because of the widespread use of carbapenem antibotics, emergence of MDR *P. aeruginosa* strains that are resistant to carbapenems has become a major concern. The rates of infections due to carbapenem-resistant *P. aeruginosa* (CRP) vary depending on geographical areas. The rates were reported to be higher in countries such as Brazil, Thailand and South Korea (14-40%) than in North America and Europe (6-20%). [37-44] Endemic countries and risk factors for infections due to CRP are shown in Table 3. Prior use of several antibiotic classes including anti-pseudomonal carbapenems, piperacillin-tazobactam, fluoroquinolones, aminoglycosides and vancomycin and other traditional risks for nosocomial infection such as presence of medical devices, prolonged hospital stay and previous colonization or infection with CRP were reported to be associated with acquisition of CRP-associated infections.

Multidrug-Resistant Acinetobacter baumannii

Acinetobacter baumannii has emerged as an important pathogen causing nosocomial infections over the last few decades. MDR *A. baumannii* isolates are usually resistant to at least 1 drug in 3 of the 6 following antibiotic classes; extended-spectrum cephalosporins, fluoroquinolones, aminoglycosides, carbapenems, piperacillin/tazobactam, and sulbactam while XDR *A. baumannii* are resistant to at least 1 drug in all antibiotic classes except colistin and tigecycline. Among *A. baumannii* isolates causing CA-UTI in the NHSN data, 78% were MDR strains and 74% were resistant to the carbapenems. [11] The increase in carbapenem-resistant *A. baumannii* (CRA)-associated infections is of global concern. Countries such as Australia, Brazil, Canada, Greece, South Korea, Spain, Taiwan and Thailand have reported CRA incidence rates of 35–80%. [45-52] Countries where CRA are endemic and risk factors for acquisition are shown in Table 3. Use of carbapenems and aminopenicillins and traditional risk factors for nosocomial infections including prolonged hospital stay, severity of illness and presence of catheters were shown to increase risk for CRA-associated infections.

Management of Multidrug-Resistant Bacterial Urinary Tract Infection

The management of MDR bacteria-associated UTIs can be categorized into 1) non-antibiotic strategies and 2) antibiotic treatment. A summary of treatment options for MDR bacteria UTIs are shown in Table 4.

Non-Antibiotic Management

Non-antibiotic strategies generally involve modification of the host status and environment to reduce the susceptibility of the host to the infection. Important measures that should be implemented include:

1. *Restoring normal urinary tract function.* To fight infection, normal urinary tract function should be restored. Patients whose active illnesses make them temporarily bed-bound, should be re-evaluated for rehabilitation and improving their mobility as soon as possible after their illnesses has improved or resolved. Maintaining of

physiologic urination in an upright or sitting position will help facilitate eradication of bacteria within the urinary tract via the urine outflow. Any causes of urinary tract obstruction, such as, nephrolithiasis and tumor and functional abnormalities of urinary tract including neurogenic bladder, reflux, and detrusor muscle dysfunction, should be evaluated by further investigations and treated accordingly.

2. *Improving host immune status.* Host immune status can be improved by 2 important measures including improving nutritional status and directly improving host immunity. Patients with MDR bacteria-associated UTIs should receive adequate and appropriate types and calories of food and protein. Appropriate nutrition is necessary for the body to maintain energy balance during the stress caused by infections and to mount a robust immune response including mobilizing polymorphonuclear cells, production of immunoglobulins, cytokines and other inflammatory mediators. The direct improvement of host immunity can be achieved depending on the underlying diseases of the patients. In patients with immunoglobulin deficiency, passive intravenous immunoglobulin is required. Decrease in or discontinuation of immunosuppressive agents, if possible, is an important strategy in patients with cancer or autoimmune disease or transplant patients who are on immunosuppressants. Antiretroviral therapy initiation, if indicated, can help restore immunity in HIV-infected patients with low CD4 cell counts. In addition, any underlying comorbidities that cause impaired immunity, such as malignancy, should be treated accordingly.
3. *Removing potential sources of urinary tract infections.* In patients with complicated UTIs, such as renal abscess or perinephric abscess, drainage of the abscess should also be performed. In patient with CA-UTIs, the indwelling catheters should be removed as soon as they are no longer required to reduce further risk of CA-UTI. [53]
4. *Implementing appropriate infection control measures.* Contact isolation should be performed for patients with or suspected to have MDR bacterial UTIs. The isolation consists of 1) placement of the patient in an isolation room or area 2) hand hygiene before and after patient contact, and after contact with patient surroundings 3) use of personal protection equipment which include gloves, gown and face mask, if indicated, when contacting the patient 4) use of dedicated medical equipment such as thermometer and stethoscope separately

for each patient and 5) clearly posting contact isolation signs and instructions in front of the patient's room or near the patient's bed. In the event that an isolation room is not available, cohorting patients with MDR bacterial infections in the same area is advisable. Implementing appropriate contact isolation and infection control measures have been demonstrated in previous studies to reduce the spread of MDR Gram-positive and Gram-negative bacteria in the healthcare settings. [54-57]

Table 4. Principle management of multidrug-resistant (MDR) bacterial urinary tract infections

Key management	Measures
Non-antibiotic management	
Restoring normal urinary tract function	Evaluating the patients for rehabilitation and early mobility Maintaining physiologic urination Correcting causes of urinary tract obstruction
Improving host immune status	Improving nutritional status Treating patients' underlying immunosuppressive diseases Decreasing the dosage of or discontinuing immunosuppressants
Removing potential source of urinary tract infection	Removing an indwelling catheter when no longer indicated Surgical intervention for complicated urinary tract infection
Implementing appropriate infection control measures	Implementing contact isolation Cohorting infected patients
Antibiotic treatment	
Administrating appropriate empiric antibiotics	Recognizing local epidemiology data and susceptibility profiles and risk factors for acquisition of MDR bacteria Early administrating the antibiotic with appropriate dose, route and interval
Administrating appropriate specific antibiotic	Adjusting antibiotic regimen according to urine culture result Early administrating the antibiotic with appropriate dose, route, interval and activity against the MDR bacteria Monitoring clinical and microbiological responses and adverse reactions of the antibiotics

Antibiotic Treatment

Antibiotic treatment can be categorized into empiric treatment and specific treatment.

1. *Empiric treatment.* Selection of empiric antibiotic treatment is based on local epidemiology data and susceptibility patterns of common uropathogens. Patients suspected to have MDR bacterial UTIs may be identified by specific risk factors associated with acquisition of each MDR Gram-positive and Gram-negative bacteria as shown in Table 2 and 3. The common risk factors include prolonged hospital stay, presence of medical devices, prior use of broad spectrum antibiotics, previous colonization or infection with MDR bacteria and being in an environment contaminated with or near a patient infected or colonized with MDR bacteria. In patients with these risk factors, empiric antibiotics that are active against MDR bacteria are necessary given that early appropriate antibiotics treatment is associated with reduced mortality. [58,59]
2. *Specific treatment.* The results of urine cultures are used to optimize antibiotic selection. Generally, factors needed to be considered for selection definite antibiotic include activity of the antibiotic against the MDR bacteria, appropriate dose, route and interval of administration based on pharmacokinetic and pharmacodynamic properties of the antibiotic, achievable drug level in the urinary tract and other co-infected sites, efficacy in prior studies and experiences in treating MDR bacterial UTIs, adverse reactions of the antibiotic, patient tolerability and cost-effectiveness. Combination treatment with at least two antibiotics from different classes or higher-than-usual dose of antibiotic is recommended if the causative bacteria are not fully susceptible or not susceptible to the antibiotics. Duration of antibiotic treatment depends on type of UTIs, systemic involvement, treatment response and related complications. Longer duration of treatment than that for non-MDR bacterial UTIs may be considered for MDR bacterial UTIs, especially in cases that there is no active antibiotic available. Generally, duration of treatment for uncomplicated lower urinary tract infection, such as cystitis, is 3-5 days for most drugs, except for forfomycin trometamol that can be given as a single dose for the treatment. [5] For acute pyelonephritis, the duration of treatment ranges from 5-14 days. Patients with acute

uncomplicated pyelonephritis without bacteremia or not requiring hospitalization can be treated for 5 days while those with bacteremia, hospitalization, immunocompromized status or that beta-lactam antibiotics are chosen as treatment regimens, duration of at least 14 days is recommended. [5, 6] For patients with complications, such as perinephric abscesses and intraabdominal infections, duration should be determined by clinical and radiological responses and be at least 14 days. [5, 7, 60] Patients who do not response to antibiotics within 3-5 days should be investigated for complications of UTIs while male patients needs to be screened for benign prostate hypertrophy, urinary tract stone or other causes of mechanical obstructions.

Specific Antibiotics for Each MDR Bacteria Causing UTIs

Antibiotics that can be used for treatment of UTIs caused by each of the MDR bacteria are shown in Table 5, 6 and 7:

Vancomycin-Resistant Enterococci

Available antibiotics that are active against VRE by the year 2013 and can be used for treatment of VRE UTIs include nitrofurantoin, daptomycin, linezolid and fosfomycin. Dose, interval, route of administration and need for dose adjustment for renal impairment are shown in Table 5. Linezolid and fosfomycin are available in both intravenous and oral forms while daptomycin is only available in intravenous form and nitrofurantoin is available in oral form only. Nitrofurantoin achieves high levels in the urinary tract and is active against VRE isolates. [61] However, it should be reserved for use in uncomplicated lower UTIs only. [5] Patient with creatinine clearance less than 40 ml/min should not be treated with nitrofurantoin due to poor renal excretion and potential accumulation of toxic metabolites. Daptomycin has good bactericidal activity against VRE and is 60% excreted in the urine in an active form. [62] In VRE UTIs with bacteremia, the dosage of 6 mg/kg should be used rather than 4 mg/kg. Linezolid is rapidly and extensively absorbed after oral dosing with an absolute bioavailability of about 100%. It is active against VRE and has cumulative renal excretion of 44% providing adequate drug level for treatment of UTIs. [62] Oral fosfomycin may be used for uncomplicated lower UTIs due to VRE while intravenous fosfomycin is preferable for acute pyelonephritis and complicated UTIs.

Table 5. Antibiotics for treatment of multidrug-resistant Gram-positive bacterial urinary tract infection (UTI)

Organism	Name of antibiotic	Route of administration	Dose and interval[a]	Renal-dose adjustment required	Important adverse reactions/comments
VRE	Nitrofurantoin	Oral	50-100 mg every 6 hours	No (Contraindicated if CrCl <60 ml/min)	Nausea, diarrhea, dizziness, fever, arthralgia, pneumonitis, hemolytic anemia Use only for uncomplicated lower UTI, such as cystitis
	Daptomycin	Intravenous	4-6 mg/kg every 24 hours	Yes	Elevated creatinine phosphokinase, insomnia, edema, headache, myopathy, rhabdomyolysis In cases with bacteremia, dose of 6 mg/kg is preferable.
	Linezolid	Oral and intravenous	600 mg every 12 hours	No	Headache, diarrhea, nausea, thrombocytopenia, lactic acidosis, peripheral neuropathy
	Fosfomycin	Oral and intravenous	Oral: 3 gram single dose Intravenous: 2 gram every 12 hours	Yes	Diarrhea, headache, nausea, dizziness, aplastic anemia, asthma exacerbation Use of oral administration is only for uncomplicated lower UTI, such as cystitis

Table 5. (Continued)

MRSA	Vancomycin	Intravenous	15-20 mg/kg every 12 hours	Yes	Red-man syndrome, nausea, rash, nephrotoxicity, ototoxicity Targeted trough level is 10-15 μg/ml. Targeted trough level is 15-20 μg/ml for coexisting bacteremia or severe infection. If MIC for vancomycin >1 μg/ml, close monitoring for clinical response is required or considering alternative antibiotics.
	Teicoplanin	Intravenous and intramuscular	400 mg loading dose followed by 200 mg daily	Yes	Injection site pain or abscess, rash, fever, dizziness, nausea, diarrhea, cross hypersensitivity with vancomycin Limited clinical data for treatment of UTI
	Daptomycin	Intravenous	4-6 mg/kg every 24 hours	Yes	Elevated creatinine phosphokinase, insomnia, edema, headache, myopathy, rhabdomyolysis In cases with bacteremia, dose of 6 mg/kg is preferable.
	Linezolid	Oral and intravenous	600 mg every 12 hours	No	Headache, diarrhea, nausea, thrombocytopenia, lactic acidosis, peripheral neuropathy
	Fosfomycin	Oral and intravenous	Oral: 3 gram single dose Intravenous: 2 gram every 12 hours	Yes	Diarrhea, headache, nausea, dizziness, aplastic anemia, asthma exacerbation Limited data for oral treatment of UTI

NOTE:[a] For patients with normal renal function

CrCl = creatinine clearance; MRSA = methicillin-resistant *Staphylococcus aureus*; VRE = vancomycin-resistant enterococci.

Table 6. Antibiotics for treatment of multidrug-resistant Enterobacteriaceae-associated Urinary Tract Infection (UTI)

Organism	Name of antibiotic	Route of administration	Dose and interval[a]	Renal-dose adjustment required	Important adverse reactions/comments
ESBL-producing Enterobacteriaceae	Imipenem	Intravenous	500 mg every 6 hours	Yes	Diarrhea, rash, nausea, hepatitis, hypersensitivity reaction
	Meropenem	Intravenous	1 gram every 8 hours	Yes	
	Doripenem	Intravenous	500 mg every 8 hours	Yes	
	Ertapenem	Intravenous and intramuscular	1 gram every 24 hours	Yes	
	Piperacillin-tazobactam	Intravenous	3.375-4.5 grams every 8 hours	Yes	Diarrhea, rash, nausea, hepatitis, headache, fever, hypersensitivity reaction
	Amoxicillin-clavulanate	Oral and intravenous	Oral: 500/125 mg or 875/125 mg every 8 hours Intravenous: 1.2 gram every 8 hours	Yes	Diarrhea, rash, nausea, hepatitis, headache, fever, hypersensitivity reaction Use of oral administration is only for uncomplicated lower UTI, such as cystitis
	Fosfomycin	Oral and intravenous	Oral: 3 gram single dose Intravenous: 2 gram every 12 hours	Yes	Diarrhea, headache, nausea, dizziness, aplastic anemia, asthma exacerbation Use of oral administration is only for uncomplicated lower UTI, such as cystitis
CRE	Colistin	Intravenous	300 mg loading followed by 150 mg every 12 hours	Yes	Dizziness, dyspepsia, paresthesia, tingling, nephrotoxicity, neurotoxicity

Table 6. (Continued)

Organism	Name of antibiotic	Route of administration	Dose and interval[a]	Renal-dose adjustment required	Important adverse reactions/comments
	Imipenem	Intravenous	1 gram drip in 3 hours every 8 hours[b]	Yes	Diarrhea, rash, nausea, hepatitis, hypersensitivity reaction Use in combination with colistin
	Meropenem	Intravenous	1 gram drip in 3 hours every 8 hours[b]	Yes	
	Doripenem	Intravenous	1 gram drip in 4 hours every 8 hours[b]	Yes	
	Gentamicin	Intravenous	5-7 mg/kg every 24 hours	Yes	Dizziness, tinnitus, nephrotoxicity, ototoxicity Use in combination with colistin Close monitoring of renal function is required, especially when combining with colistin
	Amikacin	Intravenous	15 mg/kg every 24 hours	Yes	
	Fosfomycin	Intravenous	4-6 gram drip in 4 hours every 8 hours	Yes	Diarrhea, headache, nausea, dizziness, aplastic anemia, asthma exacerbation Use in combination with colistin No data for oral treatment of UTI

NOTE:

[a] For patients with normal renal function

[b] Administration in a higher dose and prolonged infusion

CRE = carbapenem-resistant enterobacteriaceae; ESBL = extended-spectrum beta-lactamase.

Table 7. Antibiotics for treatment of carbapenem-resistant *Pseudomonas aeruginosa* (CRP)- and *Acinetobacter baumannii* (CRA)-associated urinary tract infection (UTI)

Organism	Name of antibiotic	Route of administration	Dose and interval[a]	Renal-dose adjustment required	Important adverse reactions/comments
CRP	Colistin	Intravenous	300 mg loading followed by 150 mg every 12 hours	Yes	Dizziness, dyspepsia, paresthesia, tingling, nephrotoxicity, neurotoxicity
	Imipenem	Intravenous	1 gram drip in 3 hours every 8 hours[b]	Yes	Diarrhea, rash, nausea, hepatitis, hypersensitivity reaction Use in combination with colistin
	Meropenem	Intravenous	1 gram drip in 3 hours every 8 hours[b]	Yes	
	Doripenem	Intravenous	1 gram drip in 4 hours every 8 hours[b]	Yes	
	Fosfomycin	Intravenous	4-6 grams drip in 4 hours every 8 hours	Yes	Diarrhea, headache, nausea, dizziness, aplastic anemia, asthma exacerbation
	Gentamicin	Intravenous	5-7 mg/kg every 24 hours	Yes	Dizziness, tinnitus, nephrotoxicity, ototoxicity Use in combination with colistin Close monitoring of renal function is required, especially when combining with colistin
	Amikacin	Intravenous	15 mg/kg every 24 hours	Yes	
CRA	Colistin	Intravenous	300 mg loading followed by 150 mg every 12 hours	Yes	Dizziness, dyspepsia, paresthesia, tingling, nephrotoxicity, neurotoxicity
	Imipenem	Intravenous	1 gram drip in 3 hours every 8 hours[b]	Yes	Diarrhea, rash, nausea, hepatitis, hypersensitivity reaction Use in combination with colistin
	Meropenem	Intravenous	1 gram drip in 3 hours every 8 hours[b]	Yes	

Table 7. (Continued)

Organism	Name of antibiotic	Route of administration	Dose and interval[a]	Renal-dose adjustment required	Important adverse reactions/comments
	Doripenem	Intravenous	1 gram drip in 4 hours every 8 hours[b]	Yes	
	Rifampin	Intravenous and oral	600 mg every 12 hours	No	Reddish-orange body fluid, nausea, headache, dizziness, diarrhea, cholestatic hepatitis Use in combination with colistin Close monitoring for renal function when used with colistin
	Ampicillin-sulbactam	Intravenous	Sulbactam dose of 9-12 gram per day[c]	Yes	Nausea, rash, diarrhea, hepatitis, hypersensitivity reaction
	Cefoperazole-sulbactam	Intravenous	Sulbactam dose of 6 gram per day[c]	Yes	Nausea, rash, diarrhea, hepatitis, hypersensitivity reaction

NOTE:
[a] For patients with normal renal function
[b] Administration in a higher dose and prolonged infusion
[c] The dose of sulbactam is limited by the maximal dose per day of ampicillin and cefoperazone.

In one study, 86% of VRE isolates were shown to be susceptible to fosfomycin and about 70% of the patients with VRE UTIs achieved microbiological cure. [63] However, large scale studies on clinical efficacy of fosfomycin for treatment of VRE UTI are limited.

Methicillin-Resistant Staphylococcus aureus

Available antibiotics that are active against MRSA by the year 2013 that can be used for treatment of UTIs are vancomycin, teicoplanin, daptomycin, linezolid and fosfomycin. Dose, interval, route of administration and need for dose adjustment for renal impairment of these antibiotics are shown in Table 5. Vancomycin has been the mainstay antibiotic for MRSA-related infections including UTIs for the past decades while other antibiotics should be considered when patients are intolerant of vancomycin or the infecting MRSA isolate has a high vancomycin minimum inhibitory concentration (MIC). Monitoring of vancomycin trough level during therapy is essential given that the trough level is predictive of both efficacy and toxicity. [64] For MRSA isolates with MIC $\leq$ 1 μg/ml, the effective trough level is 10-15 μg/ml for mild to moderate MRSA infections, such as skin and skin structure infection and UTI while the effective trough level is 15-20 μg/ml for more severe and complicated infections, such as bacteremia, endocarditis, endovascular infection, bone and joint infection and pneumonia. MRSA isolates with MIC $\leq$ 2 μg/ml are generally considered susceptible to vancomycin. However, multiple studies have demonstrated that vancomycin therapy in patients with severe infections, such as bacteremia and endocarditis, caused by susceptible MRSA isolates with MIC between 1.5-2 μg/ml resulted in more unfavorable outcomes than those infected with susceptible MRSA isolates with MIC less than 1.5 μg/ml. [65] Thus, in patients infected with MRSA with elevated MIC levels, close monitoring for clinical response during vancomycin therapy is essential and alternative MRSA-active agents should be considered in severe and life-threatening infections. Teicoplanin is active in-vitro against MRSA isolates. It readily penetrates tissues and achieves high level in kidneys and urinary tract. [66] However, clinical studies on the efficacy of teicoplanin in treatment of MRSA-associated UTIs are limited. A study published in 1989 revealed an overall 93% response rate for teicoplanin in treatment of MRSA-associated infections including UTIs. [67] Daptomycin is a lipopeptide antibiotic with bactericidal activity against MRSA and achieves a high urinary concentration. It has good in-vitro activity in comparison to linezolid and vancomycin for Gram-positive uropathogens causing complicated UTIs. [68] However, further clinical studies are needed to confirm the efficacy of daptomycin in treatment of MRSA-associated UTI. Linezolid is an oxazolidinone antibiotic that demonstrates good in-vitro activity against Gram-positive uropathogens including MRSA. [69] A clinical study of MRSA infections inclusive of UTIs revealed a comparable clinical and microbiological response between linezolid and vancomycin. [70] Nonetheless, specific studies on treatment of MRSA UTIs are required to confirm the clinical efficacy of linezolid. Fosfomycin demonstrates good in-vitro activity against MRSA isolates and theoretically can be used for MRSA-associated UTIs. [71] Fosfomycin is currently only approved in the US for the treatment of cystitis due to *E. coli* and enterococci and there are limited clinical data on treatment of MRSA UTIs. Oral administration of fosfomycin in uncomplicated cystitis caused by MRSA and the intravenous administration for more serious or bacteremic UTIs needs further investigations in clinical trials.

Extended-Spectrum Beta-Lactamase-Producing Enterobacteriaceae

Data on efficacy of antibiotics in the treatment of ESBL-associated infections come from small and non-randomized clinical studies. The results of these studies indicate that carbapenems were superior than other comparator drugs for treatment of ESBL infections. [72-75] Currently available and commonly used carbapenem antibiotics include imipenem, meropenem, doripenem and ertapenem. All of these carbapenems are approved for treatment of ESBL-associated UTI. However, the older carbapenems, such as imipenem and meropenem, have been studied and used more extensively than the newer carbapenems, such as ertapenem and doripenem. All of the carbapenems need to be administered intravenously and frequently each day except for ertapenem which can be given either intravenously or intramuscularly once daily. Non-carbapenem antibiotics may be used as alternatives for the treatment of ESBL-associated UTIs only if the ESBL-producing bacteria are susceptible to these agents. Such antibiotics include beta-lactamase inhibitor combinations, such as piperacillin-tazobactam and amoxicillin-clavulanate. [76,77] Fosfomycin has a good in-vitro activity against ESBL-producing Enterobacteriaceae. [78] A study from Spain demonstrated a 93% cure rate in patients with ESBL-producing *E.coli*-associated cystitis while another study from the US revealed 57% microbiological cure rate for patients with ESBL-associated UTIs treated with fosfomycin. [63,79] Well-designed clinical studies on the efficacy and outcome of fosfomycin therapy for ESBL-associated UTIs are needed. Given that there is more extensive data on the efficacy of carbapenems particularly for complicated infections, carbapenems should be considered as first-line therapy in patients with severe and/or life threatening ESBL-associated UTIs while piperacillin-tazobactam, amoxicillin-clavulanate and fosfomycin may be used as alternatives for less severe UTIs if the causative pathogens are susceptible to these antibiotics. Table 6 summarizes antibiotics for treatment of ESBL-associated UTIs.

Carbapenem-Resistant Enterobacteriaceae

There have been no well-designed randomized studies on efficacy of antibiotics for the treatment of CRE-associated infections. [80] A systematic evaluation of CRE therapy demonstrated that colistin was commonly used as monotherapy or in combination with tigecycline or carbapenem. [80] However, tigecycline is not a suitable option for UTIs given the low achievable levels in the kidneys and urinary tract. Colistin is an old polymyxin antibiotic that has recently been increasingly used for the treatment of MDR Gram-negative infections. It shows a good in-vitro activity against CRE including KPC and NDM-1-producing strains. [32,81] The commonly used formulation is colistin methanesulfonate with 2 different quantity units, milligram and international unit (1 mg equals 12,500 international units). Two systemic review of retrospective, case-control or prospective observational studies reveal that mortality rates associated with colistin monotherapy for CRE infections ranged from 27-67%. [80,82] Another treatment option is to combine colistin with other antibiotics which demonstrate in-vitro synergistic activity. These antibiotics include imipenem, fosfomycin and the aminoglycosides. [83-85] For carbapenems and fosfomycin, higher doses and administration using prolonged infusions are required to overcome the resistance of CRE. [82] Monotherapy for UTIs with an aminoglycoside, if susceptible may be appropriate given the high renal excretion but does carry with it the risk of nephrotoxicity. Fosfomycin exhibits good in-vitro activity against CRE isolates and achieves high concentration in the urine. [82,86] Limited data exists to support of use of fosfomycin as monotherapy for treatment of CRE-associated UTIs given the potential development of resistance over time during therapy. Due to the mortality benefit shown in a systemic evaluation study, combination antibiotic treatment, such as colistin and carbapenem, colistin and fosfomycin may be considered in severely ill patients with UTIs. [82] Antibiotics and their doses, methods of administration and common adverse reactions for treatment of CRE-associated UTI are shown in Table 6.

Multidrug-Resistant Pseudomonas aeruginosa

Treatment of MDR *P. aeruginosa isolates* should be guided by the results of susceptibility testing, achievable drug levels in the urinary tract system and patient characteristics. The groups of antibiotics that can be considered include 1) antipseudomonal cephalosporins, such as ceftazidime, cefepime, cefoperazone-sulbactam 2) antipseudomomal penicillins and beta-lactamase inhibitors, such as piperacillin-tazobactam 3) antipseudomonal carbapenems, such as imipenem, meropenem and doripenem 4) antipseudomonal fluoroquinolones, such as ciprofloxacin and levofloxacin 5) aminoglycosides, such as gentamicin, tobramycin and amikacin 6) aztreonam 7) fosfomycin and 8) colistin. For CRP-associated UTIs, the antibiotic options are limited and include colistin with or without a carbapenem and fosfomycin (Table 7). Colistin remains active in-vitro against most of the CRP isolates. Monotherapy with colistin has been used successfully for the treatment of CRP-associated pneumonia. [87] However, efficacy data of colistin monotherapy on CRP-associated UTI is lacking. Fosfomycin monotherapy is not recommended for treatment of any *P. aeruginosa* infections given the potential rapid development of resistance during therapy. [88] The success of combination therapy with colistin and fosfomycin or the carbapenems has been demonstrated for treatment of CRP-associated pneumonia. [89] It should be noted that both fosfomycin and the carbapenems should be administered at high doses and using an extended infusion to overcome the high MICs of CRP (Table 7). [89-91] Use of aminoglycoside monotherapy may be an option if CRP is susceptible to the aminoglycosides while the regimen combining aminoglycosides with colistin requires close monitoring for toxicity. Treatment of PDR-*P. aeruginosa*-associated UTI is difficult and challenging given no available active antibiotic options. Combination therapy is therefore an important strategy and should be based on combination antibiotic regimens that demonstrate in-vitro synergy. Such regimens include carbapenems (high dose and extended infusion) plus one of the following antibiotics: 1) colistin and rifampin, 2) fluoroquinolones and ceftazidime or cefepime and 3) ceftazidime and colistin. [92-94]

Multidrug-Resistant Acinetobacter baumannii

Antibiotic regimens for the treatment of MDR *A. baumannii*-associated UTIs can be chosen from the following groups; 1) carbapenems 2) aminoglycosides 3) sulbactam (in single drug formulation or in combination with beta-lactams, such as ampicillin-sulbactam and cefoperazone-sulbactam) 4) colistin and 5) rifampin. For CRA-associated UTIs, limited treatment options are available. Given the good in-vitro activity of colistin against CRA, treating CRA-associated infections with colistin-based regimens, either as monotherapy or in combination with other CRA-active antibiotics is a common practice. [95-98] Intravenous colistin alone resulted in a 60% success rate in treatment of CRA-associated ventilator-associated pneumonia (VAP) in a study from Greece. [99] Monotherapy with other CRA-active antibiotics has rarely been studied. Only one study demonstrated a 62% success rate using high dose amplicillin-sulbactam monotherapy for treatment of CRA-associated VAP. [99] There have been no specific published studies on the efficacy of colistin monotherapy for CRA-associated UTIs. Colistin use in combination with other available antibiotics with potential synergy such as, rifampin, sulbactam, and the carbapenems is also an option. [96-98] However, only the combination of colistin and rifampin has been studied in comparison to colistin alone. Two studies indicate that the mortality rates were not significantly different between colistin and colistin combined with rifampin but the combination regimen resulted in significantly better rates and shorter time to microbiological eradication. [95,100] Dosage, administration route and interval and adverse reactions of antibiotics for CRA are shown in Table 7. For sulbactam and carbapenems, high dose and/or extended infusion administration are required.

Conclusion

Multidrug-resistant bacterial UTIs have emerged as a major healthcare threat worldwide. Recognition of the epidemiology of these MDR Gram-positive and Gram-negative bacteria as well as patient characteristics and risk factors for acquiring such infections is crucial in selecting early and appropriate treatment for the infected patients and strategies to control the spread of these organisms. Antibiotic treatment along with non-antibiotic strategies including restoring normal urinary tract function, improving host immune status, removing potential sources of urinary tract infections such as indwelling foley catheters and implementing appropriate infection control measures are essential key components for successful management of patients with MDR bacterial UTIs.

References

[1] Apisarnthanarak A, Hsu LY, Khawcharoenporn T, Mundy LM. Carbapenem-resistant Gram-negative bacteria: how to prioritize infection prevention and control interventions in resource-limited settings? *Expert Rev. Anti Infect. Ther.* 2013; 11: 147-57.

[2] Lautenbach E, Weiner MG, Nachamkin I, Bilker WB, Sheridan A, Fishman NO. Imipenem resistance among *Pseudomonas aeruginosa* isolates: risk factors for infection and impact of resistance on clinical and economic outcomes. *Infect. Control Hosp. Epidemiol.* 2006; 27: 893-900.

[3] Sheng WH, Liao CH, Lauderdale TL, et al. A multicenter study of risk factors and outcome of hospitalized patients with infections due to carbapenem-resistant *Acinetobacter baumannii*. *Int. J. Infect. Dis.* 2010; 14: e764-9.

[4] Schwaber MJ, Klarfeld-Lidji S, Navon-Venezia S, Schwartz D, Leavitt A, Carmeli Y. Predictors of carbapenem-resistant *Klebsiella pneumoniae* acquisition among hospitalized adults and effect of acquisition on mortality. *Antimicrob. Agents Chemother* 2008; 52: 1028-33.

[5] Gupta K, Hooton TM, Naber KG, et al. International clinical practice guidelines for the treatment of acute uncomplicated cystitis and pyelonephritis in women: A 2010 update by the Infectious Diseases Society of America and the European Society for Microbiology and Infectious Diseases. *Clin. Infect. Dis.* 2011; 52: e103-20.

[6] Hooton TM, Bradley SF, Cardenas DD, et al. Diagnosis, prevention, and treatment of catheter-associated urinary tract infection in adults: 2009 International Clinical Practice Guidelines from the Infectious Diseases Society of America. *Clin. Infect. Dis.* 2010; 50: 625-63.

[7] Nicolle LE. Complicated urinary tract infection in adults. *Can. J. Infect. Dis. Med. Microbiol.* 2005; 16: 349-60.

[8] Hooton TM. Uncomplicated urinary tract infection. *N. Engl. J. Med.* 2012; 366: 1028-37.

[9] Magiorakos AP, Srinivasan A, Carey RB, et al. Multidrug-resistant, extensively drug-resistant and pandrug-resistant bacteria: an international expert proposal for interim standard definitions for acquired resistance. *Clin. Microbiol. Infect.* 2012; 18: 268-81.

[10] Zhanel GG, Hisanaga TL, Laing NM, et al. Antibiotic resistance in outpatient urinary isolates: final results from the North American Urinary Tract Infection Collaborative Alliance (NAUTICA). *Int. J. Antimicrob. Agents* 2005; 26: 380-8.

[11] Sievert DM, Ricks P, Edwards JR, et al. Antimicrobial-resistant pathogens associated with healthcare-associated infections: summary of data reported to the National Healthcare Safety Network at the Centers for Disease Control and Prevention, 2009-2010. *Infect. Control Hosp. Epidemiol.* 2013; 34: 1-14.

[12] Song JH, Hsueh PR, Chung DR, et al. Spread of methicillin-resistant *Staphylococcus aureus* between the community and the hospitals in Asian countries: an ANSORP study. *J. Antimicrob. Chemother.* 2011; 66: 1061-9.

[13] MacDougall C, Powell JP, Johnson CK, Edmond MB, Polk RE. Hospital and community fluoroquinolone use and resistance in *Staphylococcus aureus* and *Escherichia coli* in 17 US hospitals. *Clin. Infect. Dis.* 2005; 41: 435-40.

[14] Hill DA, Herford T, Parratt D. Antibiotic usage and methicillin-resistant *Staphylococcus aureus*: an analysis of causality. *J. Antimicrob. Chemother.* 1998; 42: 676-7.

[15] Centers for Disease Control and Prevention (CDC). Invasive methicillin-resistant *Staphylococcus aureus* infections among dialysis patients--United States, 2005. *MMWR Morb. Mortal Wkly Rep.* 2007; 56: 197-9.

[16] Thompson RL, Cabezudo I, Wenzel RP. Epidemiology of nosocomial infections caused by methicillin-resistant *Staphylococcus aureus. Ann. Intern. Med.* 1982; 97: 309-17.

[17] Boyce JM. Methicillin-resistant *Staphylococcus aureus.* Detection, epidemiology, and control measures. *Infect. Dis. Clin. North Am.* 1989; 3: 901-13.

[18] Davis KA, Stewart JJ, Crouch HK, Florez CE, Hospenthal DR. Methicillin-resistant *Staphylococcus aureus* (MRSA) nares colonization at hospital admission and its effect on subsequent MRSA infection. *Clin. Infect. Dis.* 2004; 39: 776-82.

[19] Diep BA, Chambers HF, Graber CJ, et al. Emergence of multidrug-resistant, community-associated, methicillin-resistant *Staphylococcus aureus* clone USA300 in men who have sex with men. *Ann. Intern. Med.* 2008; 148: 249-57.

[20] Byrd KK, Holman RC, Bruce MG, et al. Methicillin-resistant *Staphylococcus aureus*-associated hospitalizations among the American Indian and Alaska native population. *Clin. Infect. Dis.* 2009; 49: 1009-15.

[21] Centers for Disease Control and Prevention (CDC). Methicillin-resistant *Staphylococcus aureus* infections among competitive sports participants--Colorado, Indiana, Pennsylvania, and Los Angeles County, 2000-2003. *MMWR Morb. Mortal Wkly Rep.* 2003; 52: 793-5.

[22] Aiello AE, Lowy FD, Wright LN, Larson EL. Meticillin-resistant *Staphylococcus aureus* among US prisoners and military personnel: review and recommendations for future studies. *Lancet Infect. Dis.* 2006; 6: 335-41.

[23] Centers for Disease Control and Prevention. Public health dispatch: outbreaks of community-associated methicillin-resistant *Staphylococcus aureus* skin infections--Los Angeles County, California, 2002-2003. JAMA 2003; 289: 1377.

[24] Khawcharoenporn T, Vasoo S, Singh K. Urinary tract infections due to multidrug-resistant Enterobacteriaceae: prevalence and risk Factors in a Chicago Emergency Department. *Emerg. Med. Int.* 2013;2013:258517. [Epub ahead of print].

[25] Lu PL, Liu YC, Toh HS, et al. Epidemiology and antimicrobial susceptibility profiles of Gram-negative bacteria causing urinary tract infections in the Asia-Pacific region: 2009-2010 results from the Study for Monitoring Antimicrobial Resistance Trends (SMART). *Int. J. Antimicrob. Agents* 2012; 40 Suppl: S37-43.

[26] Bours PH, Polak R, Hoepelman AI, et al. Increasing resistance in community-acquired urinary tract infections in Latin America, five years after the implementation of national therapeutic guidelines. *Int. J. Infect. Dis.* 2010; 14: e770-4.

[27] Kothari A, Sagar V. Antibiotic resistance in pathogens causing community-acquired urinary tract infections in India: a multicenter study. *J. Infect. Dev. Ctries* 2008; 2: 354-8.

[28] Jacoby GA, Munoz-Price LS. The new beta-lactamases. *N. Engl. J. Med.* 2005; 352: 380-91.

[29] Jacoby GA. Epidemiology of extended-spectrum beta-lactamases. *Clin. Infect. Dis.* 1998; 27: 81-3.

[30] Paterson DL, Ko WC, Von Gottberg A, et al. International prospective study of *Klebsiella pneumoniae* bacteremia: implications of extended-spectrum beta-lactamase production in nosocomial infections. *Ann. Intern. Med.* 2004; 140: 26-32.

[31] Apisarnthanarak A, Hsu LY, Khawcharoenporn T, Mundy LM. Carbapenem-resistant Gram-negative bacteria: how to prioritize infection prevention and control interventions in resource-limited settings? *Expert Rev. Anti Infect. Ther.* 2013; 11: 147-57.

[32] Kumarasamy KK, Toleman MA, Walsh TR et al. Emergence of a new antibiotic resistance mechanism in India, Pakistan, and the UK: a molecular, biological, and epidemiological study. *Lancet Infect. Dis.* 2010; 10: 597–602.

[33] Vatopoulos A. High rates of metallo-β-lactamase-producing *Klebsiella pneumoniae* in Greece – a review of the current evidence. *Euro Surveill* 2008; 13: 8023.

[34] Hidron AI, Edwards JR, Patel J et al. National Healthcare Safety Network Team; Participating National Healthcare Safety Network Facilities. NHSN annual update: antimicrobial-resistant pathogens associated with healthcare-associated infections: annual summary of data reported to the National Healthcare Safety Network at the Centers for Disease Control and Prevention, 2006–2007. *Infect. Control Hosp. Epidemiol.* 2008; 29: 996–1011.

[35] Rhomberg PR, Jones RN. Summary trends for the Meropenem Yearly Susceptibility Test Information Collection Program: a 10-year experience in the United States (1999–2008). *Diagn. Microbiol. Infect. Dis.* 2009; 65: 414–26.

[36] Bratu S, Landman D, Haag R et al. Rapid spread of carbapenem-resistant *Klebsiella pneumoniae* in New York City: a new threat to our antibiotic armamentarium. *Arch. Intern. Med.* 2005; 165: 1430–5.

[37] Baumgart AM, Molinari MA, Silveira AC. Prevalence of carbapenem resistant *Pseudomonas aeruginosa* and *Acinetobacter baumannii* in high complexity hospital. *Braz. J. Infect. Dis.* 2010; 14: 433–6.

[38] Dejsirilert S, Suankratay C, Trakulsomboon S et al. National Antimicrobial Resistance Surveillance, Thailand (NARST) data among clinical isolates of *Pseudomonas aeruginosa* in Thailand from 2000 to 2005. *J. Med. Assoc. Thai.* 2009; 92: S68–75.

[39] Behera B, Das A, Mathur P, Kapil A. High prevalence of carbapenem resistant *Pseudomonas aeruginosa* at a tertiary-care center of north India. Are we under-reporting? *Indian J. Med. Res.* 2008; 128: 324–5.

[40] Lee JY, Ko KS. OprD mutations and inactivation, expression of efflux pumps and AmpC, and metallo-β-lactamases in carbapenem-resistant *Pseudomonas aeruginosa* isolates from South Korea. *Int. J. Antimicrob. Agents* 2012; 40: 168–72.

[41] Onguru P, Erbay A, Bodur H et al. Imipenem-resistant *Pseudomonas aeruginosa*: risk factors for nosocomial infections. *J. Korean Med. Sci.* 2008; 23: 982–7.

[42] Rhomberg PR, Deshpande LM, Kirby JT, Jones RN. Activity of meropenem as serine carbapenemases evolve in US Medical Centers: monitoring report from the MYSTIC Program (2006). *Diagn. Microbiol. Infect. Dis.* 2007; 59: 425–32.

[43] Harris AD, Smith D, Johnson JA, Bradham DD, Roghmann MC. Risk factors for imipenem-resistant *Pseudomonas aeruginosa* among hospitalized patients. *Clin. Infect. Dis.* 2002; 34: 340-5.

[44] Lagatolla C, Tonin EA, Monti-Bragadin C et al. Endemic carbapenem-resistant *Pseudomonas aeruginosa* with acquired metallo-β-lactamase determinants in European hospital. *Emerging. Infect. Dis.* 2004; 10: 535–8.

[45] Peleg AY, Franklin C, Bell JM, Spelman DW. Emergence of carbapenem resistance in *Acinetobacter baumannii* recovered from blood cultures in Australia. *Infect. Control Hosp. Epidemiol.* 2006; 27: 759–61.

[46] Baumgart AM, Molinari MA, Silveira AC. Prevalence of carbapenem resistant *Pseudomonas aeruginosa* and *Acinetobacter baumannii* in high complexity hospital. *Braz. J. Infect. Dis.* 2010; 14: 433–6.

[47] Mataseje LF, Bryce E, Roscoe D et al. Canadian Nosocomial Infection Surveillance Program. Carbapenem-resistant Gram-negative bacilli in Canada 2009–10: results from the Canadian Nosocomial Infection Surveillance Program (CNISP). *J. Antimicrob. Chemother.* 2012; 67: 1359–67.

[48] Ying CM, Ling TK, Lee CC, Ling JM. Characterization of carbapenem-resistant *Acinetobacter baumannii* in Shanghai and Hong Kong. *J. Med. Microbiol.* 2006; 55: 799–802.

[49] Kim YJ, Kim SI, Kim YR et al. Carbapenem-resistant *Acinetobacter baumannii*: diversity of resistant mechanisms and risk factors for infection. *Epidemiol. Infect.* 2012; 140: 137–45.

[50] Asensio A, Cantón R, Vaqué J et al. Prevalence of infection by carbapenem-resistant *Acinetobacter baumannii* in Spain (1999–2005). *Enferm. Infecc. Microbiol. Clin.* 2008; 26: 199–204.

[51] Sheng WH, Liao CH, Lauderdale TL et al. A multicenter study of risk factors and outcome of hospitalized patients with infections due to carbapenem-resistant *Acinetobacter baumannii*. *Int. J. Infect. Dis.* 2010; 14: e764–9.

[52] Dejsirilert S, Tiengrim S, Sawanpanyalert P, Aswapokee N, Malathum K. Antimicrobial resistance of *Acinetobacter baumannii*: six years of National Antimicrobial Resistance Surveillance Thailand (NARST) surveillance. *J. Med. Assoc. Thai.* 2009; 92: S34–45.

[53] Hooton TM, Bradley SF, Cardenas DD, et al. Diagnosis, prevention, and treatment of catheter-associated urinary tract infection in adults: 2009 international clinical practice guidelines from the Infectious Diseases Society of America. *Clin. Infect. Dis.* 2010; 50: 625–63.

[54] Puzniak LA, Leet T, Mayfield J, Kollef M, Mundy LM. To gown or not to gown: the effect on acquisition of vancomycin-resistant enterococci. *Clin. Infect. Dis.* 2002; 35: 18-25.

[55] Muto CA, Jernigan JA, Ostrowsky BE, et al. SHEA guideline for preventing nosocomial transmission of multidrug-resistant strains of *Staphylococcus aureus* and enterococcus. *Infect. Control Hosp. Epidemiol.* 2003; 24: 362-86.

[56] Lucet JC, Decré D, Fichelle A, et al. Control of a prolonged outbreak of extended-spectrum beta-lactamase-producing Enterobacteriaceae in a university hospital. *Clin. Infect. Dis.* 1999; 29: 1411-8.

[57] Kochar S, Sheard T, Sharma R, et al. Success of an infection control program to reduce the spread of carbapenem-resistant *Klebsiella pneumoniae*. *Infect. Control Hosp. Epidemiol.* 2009; 30: 447-52.

[58] Paterson DL, Ko WC, Von Gottberg A, et al. Antibiotic therapy for *Klebsiella pneumoniae* bacteremia: implications of production of extended-spectrum beta-lactamases. *Clin. Infect. Dis.* 2004; 39: 31-7.

[59] Zarkotou O, Pournaras S, Tselioti P, et al. Predictors of mortality in patients with bloodstream infections caused by KPC-producing *Klebsiella pneumoniae* and impact of appropriate antimicrobial treatment. *Clin. Microbiol. Infect.* 2011; 17: 1798-803.

[60] Hayashi Y, Paterson DL. Strategies for reduction in duration of antibiotic use in hospitalized patients. *Clin. Infect. Dis.* 2011; 52: 1232-40.

[61] Zhanel GG, Laing NM, Nichol KA, et al. Antibiotic activity against urinary tract infection (UTI) isolates of vancomycin-resistant enterococci (VRE): results from the 2002 North American Vancomycin Resistant Enterococci Susceptibility Study (NAVRESS). *J. Antimicrob. Chemother.* 2003; 52: 382-8.

[62] Wagenlehner FM, Naber KG. New drugs for Gram-positive uropathogens. *Int. J. Antimicrob. Agents* 2004; 24: S39-43.

[63] Neuner EA, Sekeres J, Hall GS, van Duin D. Experience with fosfomycin for treatment of urinary tract infections due to multidrug-resistant organisms. *Antimicrob. Agents Chemother.* 2012; 56: 5744-8.

[64] Rybak MJ, Lomaestro BM, Rotschafer JC, et al. Therapeutic monitoring of vancomycin in adults summary of consensus recommendations from the American Society of Health-System Pharmacists, the Infectious Diseases Society of America, and the Society of Infectious Diseases Pharmacists. *Pharmacotherapy* 2009; 29: 1275-9.

[65] Holland TL, Fowler VG Jr. Vancomycin minimum inhibitory concentration and outcome in patients with *Staphylococcus aureus* bacteremia: pearl or pellet? *J. Infect. Dis.* 2011; 204: 329-31.

[66] Sanofi-Aventis. Summary of product characteristics: Targocid. Available at: http://www.sanofi-aventis.co.uk/products/Targocid_SPC.pdf. Accessed 1 November 2013.

[67] de Lalla F, Santoro D, Rinaldi E, et al. Teicoplanin in the treatment of infections by staphylococci, *Clostridium difficile* and other gram-positive bacteria. *J. Antimicrob. Chemother.* 1989; 23: 131-42.

[68] Beiras-Fernandez A, Vogt F, Sodian R, Weis F. Daptomycin: a novel lipopeptide antibiotic against Gram-positive pathogens. *Infect. Drug Resist.* 2010; 3: 95-101.

[69] Onda H, Wagenlehner FM, Lehn N, Naber KG. In vitro activity of linezolid against Gram-positive uropathogens of hospitalized patients with complicated urinary tract infections. *Int. J. Antimicrob. Agents* 2001; 18: 263-6.

[70] Stevens DL, Herr D, Lampiris H, Hunt JL, Batts DH, Hafkin B. Linezolid versus vancomycin for the treatment of methicillin-resistant *Staphylococcus aureus* infections. *Clin. Infect. Dis.* 2002; 34: 1481-90.

[71] Lu CL, Liu CY, Huang YT, et al. Antimicrobial susceptibilities of commonly encountered bacterial isolates to fosfomycin determined by agar dilution and disk diffusion methods. *Antimicrob. Agents Chemother.* 2011; 55: 4295-301.

[72] Paterson DL, Ko WC, Von Gottberg A, et al. Antibiotic therapy for *Klebsiella pneumoniae* bacteremia: implications of production of extended-spectrum beta-lactamases. *Clin. Infect. Dis.* 2004; 39: 31-7.

[73] Bhavnani SM, Ambrose PG, Craig WA, et al. Outcomes evaluation of patients with ESBL- and non-ESBL-producing *Escherichia coli* and *Klebsiella species* as defined by CLSI reference methods: report from the SENTRY Antimicrobial Surveillance Program. *Diagn. Microbiol. Infect. Dis* 2006; 54: 231-6.

[74] Zanetti G, Bally F, Greub G, et al. Cefepime versus imipenem-cilastatin for treatment of nosocomial pneumonia in intensive care unit patients: a multicenter, evaluator-blind, prospective, randomized study. *Antimicrob. Agents Chemother.* 2003; 47: 3442-7.

[75] Vardakas KZ, Tansarli GS, Rafailidis PI, Falagas ME. Carbapenems versus alternative antibiotics for the treatment of bacteraemia due to Enterobacteriaceae producing extended-spectrum β-lactamases: a systematic review and meta-analysis. *J. Antimicrob. Chemother.* 2012; 67: 2793-803.

[76] Gavin PJ, Suseno MT, Thomson RB Jr, et al. Clinical correlation of the CLSI susceptibility breakpoint for piperacillin-tazobactam against extended-spectrum-beta-lactamase-producing *Escherichia coli* and *Klebsiella* species. *Antimicrob. Agents Chemother.* 2006; 50: 2244-7.

[77] Rodríguez-Baño J, Navarro MD, Retamar P, et al. β-Lactam/β-lactam inhibitor combinations for the treatment of bacteremia due to extended-spectrum β-lactamase-producing *Escherichia coli*: a post hoc analysis of prospective cohorts. *Clin. Infect. Dis.* 2012; 54: 167-74.

[78] de Cueto M, López L, Hernández JR, Morillo C, Pascual A. In vitro activity of fosfomycin against extended-spectrum-beta-lactamase-producing *Escherichia coli* and *Klebsiella pneumoniae*: comparison of susceptibility testing procedures. *Antimicrob. Agents Chemother.* 2006; 50: 368-70.

[79] Rodríguez-Baño J, Alcalá JC, Cisneros JM, et al. Community infections caused by extended-spectrum beta-lactamase-producing *Escherichia coli*. *Arch. Intern. Med.* 2008; 168: 1897-902.

[80] Falagas ME, Lourida P, Poulikakos P, Rafailidis PI, Tansarli GS. Antibiotic treatment of infections due to carbapenem-resistant Enterobacteriaceae: systematic evaluation of the available evidence. *Antimicrob. Agents Chemother.* 2013 Sep 30. [Epub ahead of print].

[81] Gupta N, Limbago BM, Patel JB, Kallen AJ. Carbapenem-Resistant Enterobacteriaceae: Epidemiology and Prevention. *Clin. Infect. Dis.* 2011; 53: 60–7.

[82] Petrosillo N, Giannella M, Lewis R, Viale P. Treatment of carbapenem-resistant *Klebsiella pneumoniae*: the state of the art. *Expert. Rev. Anti Infect. Ther.* 2013; 11: 159-77.

[83] Souli M, Rekatsina PD, Chryssouli Z, Galani I, Giamarellou H, Kanellakopoulou K. Does the activity of the combination of imipenem and colistin in vitro exceed the problem of resistance in metallo-β-

lactamase-producing *Klebsiella pneumoniae* isolates? *Antimicrob. Agents Chemother.* 2009; 53: 2133–5.

[84] Jernigan MG, Press EG, Nguyen MH, Clancy CJ, Shields RK. The combination of doripenem and colistin is bactericidal and synergistic against colistin-resistant, carbapenemase-producing *Klebsiella pneumoniae. Antimicrob. Agents Chemother.* 2012; 56: 3395–8.

[85] Samonis G, Maraki S, Karageorgopoulos DE, Vouloumanou EK, Falagas ME. Synergy of fosfomycin with carbapenems, colistin, netilmicin, and tigecycline against multidrug-resistant *Klebsiella pneumoniae*, *Escherichia coli*, and *Pseudomonas aeruginosa* clinical isolates. *Eur. J. Clin. Microbiol. Infect. Dis.* 2012; 31: 695–701.

[86] Falagas ME, Kastoris AC, Kapaskelis AM, Karageorgopoulos DE. Fosfomycin for the treatment of multidrug-resistant, including extended-spectrum β-lactamase producing, Enterobacteriaceae infections: a systematic review. *Lancet Infect. Dis.* 2010; 10; 43–50.

[87] Kwa AL, Loh C, Low JG, Kurup A, Tam VH. Nebulized colistin in the treatment of pneumonia due to multidrug-resistant *Acinetobacter baumannii* and *Pseudomonas aeruginosa. Clin. Infect. Dis.* 2005; 41: 754-7.

[88] Popovic M, Steinort D, Pillai S, Joukhadar C. Fosfomycin: an old, new friend? *Eur. J. Clin. Microbiol. Infect. Dis.* 2010; 29: 127-42.

[89] Apisarnthanarak A, Mundy LM. Use of high-dose 4-hour infusion of doripenem, in combination with fosfomycin, for treatment of carbapenem-resistant *Pseudomonas aeruginosa* pneumonia. *Clin. Infect. Dis.* 2010; 51: 1352-4.

[90] Louie A, Bied A, Fregeau C, et al. Impact of different carbapenems and regimens of administration on resistance emergence for three isogenic *Pseudomonas aeruginosa* strains with differing mechanisms of resistance. *Antimicrob Agents Chemother* 2010; 54: 2638-45.

[91] Koomanachai P, Bulik CC, Kuti JL, Nicolau DP. Pharmacodynamic modeling of intravenous antibiotics against gram-negative bacteria collected in the United States. *Clin. Ther.* 2010; 32: 766-79.

[92] Fish DN, Choi MK, Jung R. Synergic activity of cephalosporins plus fluoroquinolones against *Pseudomonas aeruginosa* with resistance to one or both drugs. *J. Antimicrob. Chemother.* 2002; 50: 1045-9.

[93] Gunderson BW, Ibrahim KH, Hovde LB, Fromm TL, Reed MD, Rotschafer JC. Synergistic activity of colistin and ceftazidime against multiantibiotic-resistant *Pseudomonas aeruginosa* in an in vitro pharmacodynamic model. *Antimicrob. Agents Chemother.* 2003; 47: 905-9.

[94] Timurkaynak F, Can F, Azap OK, Demirbilek M, Arslan H, Karaman SO. In vitro activities of non-traditional antimicrobials alone or in combination against multidrug-resistant strains of *Pseudomonas aeruginosa* and *Acinetobacter baumannii* isolated from intensive care units. *Int. J. Antimicrob. Agents* 2006; 27: 224-8.

[95] Durante-Mangoni E, Signoriello G, Andini R, et al. Colistin and rifampicin compared with colistin alone for the treatment of serious infections due to extensively drug-resistant *Acinetobacter baumannii*: a multicenter, randomized clinical trial. *Clin. Infect. Dis.* 2013; 57: 349-58.

[96] Mutlu Yilmaz E, Sunbul M, Aksoy A, Yilmaz H, Guney AK, Guvenc T. Efficacy of tigecycline/colistin combination in a pneumonia model caused by extensively drug-resistant *Acinetobacter baumannii*. *Int. J. Antimicrob. Agents* 2012; 40: 332-6.

[97] Pachón-Ibáñez ME, Docobo-Pérez F, López-Rojas R, et al. Efficacy of rifampin and its combinations with imipenem, sulbactam, and colistin in experimental models of infection caused by imipenem-resistant *Acinetobacter baumannii*. *Antimicrob. Agents Chemother.* 2010; 54: 1165-72.

[98] Pongpech P, Amornnopparattanakul S, Panapakdee S, et al. Antibacterial activity of carbapenem-based combinations againts multidrug-resistant *Acinetobacter baumannii*. *J. Med. Assoc. Thai.* 2010; 93: 161-71.

[99] Betrosian AP, Frantzeskaki F, Xanthaki A, Douzinas EE. Efficacy and safety of high-dose ampicillin/sulbactam vs. colistin as monotherapy for the treatment of multidrug resistant *Acinetobacter baumannii* ventilator-associated pneumonia. *J. Infect.* 2008; 56: 432-6.

[100] Aydemir H, Akduman D, Piskin N, et al. Colistin vs. the combination of colistin and rifampicin for the treatment of carbapenem-resistant *Acinetobacter baumannii* ventilator-associated pneumonia. *Epidemiol. Infect.* 2013; 141: 1214-22.

[101] Kang Y, Vicente M, Parsad S, et al. Evaluation of risk factors for vancomycin-resistant Enterococcus bacteremia among previously colonized hematopoietic stem cell transplant patients. *Transpl. Infect. Dis.* 2013; 15: 466-73.

[102] Vydra J, Shanley RM, George I, et al. Enterococcal bacteremia is associated with increased risk of mortality in recipients of allogeneic hematopoietic stem cell transplantation. *Clin. Infect. Dis.* 2012; 55: 764-70.

[103] Olivier CN, Blake RK, Steed LL, Salgado CD. Risk of vancomycin-resistant Enterococcus (VRE) bloodstream infection among patients colonized with VRE. *Infect. Control Hosp. Epidemiol.* 2008; 29: 404-9.

[104] Ghanem G, Hachem R, Jiang Y, Chemaly RF, Raad I. Outcomes for and risk factors associated with vancomycin-resistant *Enterococcus faecalis* and vancomycin-resistant *Enterococcus faecium* bacteremia in cancer patients. *Infect. Control Hosp. Epidemiol.* 2007; 28: 1054-9.

[105] Martínez JA, Ruthazer R, Hansjosten K, Barefoot L, Snydman DR. Role of environmental contamination as a risk factor for acquisition of vancomycin-resistant enterococci in patients treated in a medical intensive care unit. *Arch. Intern. Med.* 2003; 163: 1905-12.

[106] Carmeli Y, Eliopoulos GM, Samore MH. Antecedent treatment with different antibiotic agents as a risk factor for vancomycin-resistant Enterococcus. *Emerg. Infect. Dis.* 2002; 8: 802-7.

[107] Dahms RA, Johnson EM, Statz CL, Lee JT, Dunn DL, Beilman GJ. Third-generation cephalosporins and vancomycin as risk factors for postoperative vancomycin-resistant Enterococcus infection. *Arch. Surg.* 1998; 133: 1343-6.

[108] Furtado GH, Mendes RE, Pignatari AC, Wey SB, Medeiros EA. Risk factors for vancomycin-resistant *Enterococcus faecalis* bacteremia in hospitalized patients: an analysis of two case-control studies. *Am. J. Infect. Control* 2006; 34: 447-51.

[109] Popovich KJ, Weinstein RA, Aroutcheva A, Rice T, Hota B. Community-associated methicillin-resistant *Staphylococcus aureus* and HIV: intersecting epidemics. *Clin. Infect. Dis.* 2010; 50: 979-87.

[110] Mathews WC, Caperna JC, Barber RE, et al. Incidence of and risk factors for clinically significant methicillin-resistant *Staphylococcus aureus* infection in a cohort of HIV-infected adults. *J. Acquir. Immune. Defic. Syndr.* 2005; 40: 155-60.

[111] Mataseje LF, Bryce E, Roscoe D et al. Canadian Nosocomial Infection Surveillance Program. Carbapenem-resistant Gram-negative bacilli in Canada 2009–10: results from the Canadian Nosocomial Infection Surveillance Program (CNISP). *J. Antimicrob. Chemother.* 2012; 67: 1359–67.

[112] Patel G, Huprikar S, Factor SH, Jenkins SG, Calfee DP. Outcomes of carbapenem-resistant *Klebsiella pneumoniae* infection and the impact of antimicrobial and adjunctive therapies. *Infect. Control Hosp. Epidemiol.* 2008; 29: 1099–106.

[113] Hussein K, Sprecher H, Mashiach T, Oren I, Kassis I, Finkelstein R. Carbapenem resistance among *Klebsiella pneumoniae* isolates: risk factors, molecular characteristics, and susceptibility patterns. *Infect. Control Hosp. Epidemiol.* 2009; 30: 666–71.

[114] Wu D, Cai J, Liu J. Risk factors for the acquisition of nosocomial infection with carbapenem-resistant *Klebsiella pneumoniae*. *South. Med. J.* 2011; 104: 106–10.

[115] Jeon MH, Choi SH, Kwak YG et al. Risk factors for the acquisition of carbapenem-resistant *Escherichia coli* among hospitalized patients. *Diagn. Microbiol. Infect. Dis.* 2008; 62: 402–6.

[116] Mouloudi E, Protonotariou E, Zagorianou A et al. Bloodstream infections caused by metallo-b-lactamase/*Klebsiella pneumoniae* carbapenemase-producing *K. pneumoniae* among intensive care unit patients in Greece: risk factors for infection and impact of type of resistance on outcomes. *Infect. Control Hosp. Epidemiol.* 2010; 31: 1250–6.

[117] Kohlenberg A, Weitzel-Kage D, van der Linden P et al. Outbreak of carbapenem-resistant *Pseudomonas aeruginosa* infection in a surgical intensive care unit. *J. Hosp. Infect.* 2010; 74: 350–7.

[118] Peña C, Suarez C, Tubau F et al. Carbapenem-resistant *Pseudomonas aeruginosa*: factors influencing multidrug-resistant acquisition in non-critically ill patients. *Eur. J. Clin. Microbiol. Infect. Dis.* 2009; 28: 519–22.

[119] Ozkurt Z, Ertek M, Erol S, Altoparlak U, Akcay MN. The risk factors for acquisition of imipenem-resistant *Pseudomonas aeruginosa* in the burn unit. *Burns* 2005; 31: 870–3.

[120] BA. Zavascki AP, Cruz RP, Goldani LZ. Risk factors for imipenem-resistant *Pseudomonas aeruginosa*: a comparative analysis of two case–control studies in hospitalized patients. *J. Hosp. Infect.* 2005; 59: 96–101.

[121] Furtado GH, Gales AC, Perdiz LB, Santos AE, Wey SB, Medeiros EA. Risk factors for hospital-acquired pneumonia caused by imipenem-resistant *Pseudomonas aeruginosa* in an intensive care unit. *Anaesth. Intensive Care* 2010; 38: 994–1001.

[122] Le Hello S, Falcot V, Lacassin F, Mikulski M, Baumann F. Risk factors for carbapenem-resistant *Acinetobacter baumannii* infections at a tertiary care hospital in New Caledonia, South Pacific. *Scand. J. Infect. Dis.* 2010; 42: 821–6.

[123] Akinci E, Colpan A, Bodur H, Balaban N, Erbay A. Risk factors for ICU-acquired imipenem-resistant Gram-negative bacterial infections. *J. Hosp. Infect.* 2005; 59: 317–23.

[124] Playford EG, Craig JC, Iredell JR. Carbapenem-resistant *Acinetobacter baumannii* in intensive care unit patients: risk factors for acquisition, infection and their consequences. *J Hosp Infect*; 2007: 65: 204–11.

Index

B

C

D

E

F

G

H

K

L

M

N

R

S

T

U

V

W

Y